FAT FLUSH FOR LIFE

FAT FLUSH FOR LIFE

The Year-Round Super
Detox Plan to Boost Your
Metabolism and Keep the
Weight Off Permanently

Ann Louise Gittleman, PhD, CNS

Da Capo
LIFE
LONG

A Member of the
Perseus Books Group

Design and production by Dean R. Howes

Cataloging-in-Publication data for this book is available from the Library of Congress.

First Da Capo Press edition 2010
ISBN: 978-0-7382-1366-8

Published by Da Capo Press
A Member of the Perseus Books Group
www.dacapopress.com

Note: The information in this book is true and complete to the best of our knowledge. This book is intended only as an informative guide for those wishing to know more about health issues. In no way is this book intended to replace, countermand, or conflict with the advice given to you by your own physician. The ultimate decision concerning care should be made between you and your doctor. We strongly recommend you follow his or her advice. Information in this book is general and is offered with no guarantees on the part of the authors or Da Capo Press. The authors and publisher disclaim all liability in connection with the use of this book. The names and identifying details of people associated with events described in this book have been changed. Any similarity to actual persons is coincidental.

Da Capo Press books are available at special discounts for bulk purchases in the U.S. by corporations, institutions, and other organizations. For more information, please contact the Special Markets Department at the Perseus Books Group, 2300 Chestnut Street, Suite 200, Philadelphia, PA, 19103, or call (800) 810-4145, ext. 5000, or e-mail special.markets@ perseusbooks.com.

10 9 8 7 6 5 4 3 2 1

For Linda . . .

Contents

Acknowledgments

As a little girl, I was taught that two unseen angels accompany every human being at birth. But, for some reason, I have been blessed with a special band of angels in the form of my family members, friends, associates, editors, volunteers, and assorted healers, who have made this book possible.

I am very indebted to the entire Da Capo team, especially Katie McHugh, my executive editor, for her enlightened vision and direction. Thanks also to Katie's assistants, Wesley Royce and Erica Truxler, and especially to Cisca L. Schreefel, the senior project editor whose expertise made my job a pleasure in the final stages. Blessings on the head of Sue McCloskey, who so effortlessly helped to transform this manuscript with her editorial know-how and grace. Many thanks to the rest of the Da Capo team—Julia Hall; Wendy Carr, publicist extraordinaire; and Iris Bass—for all their help.

My agent, the indefatigable Coleen O'Shea, is to be congratulated for continuing to be my greatest fan and a bastion of common sense and voice of "reason." Coleen always knows best! My profound thanks to Stuart Gittleman, my significant brother, for his operational skills in seeing that First Lady of Nutrition was operating at peak proficiency while I was writing and rewriting for so many months. Everybody should be so lucky, whether personally or professionally, to have a Stuart!

Thank you to Carol Templeton for her contagious enthusiasm. Major kudos to Linda Mitchell, who collaborated with me on the fitness sections, and her daughter, Tiffany Nicholson, whose photos of her mom are beautiful as well as instructive. Heartfelt thanks to Linda Shapiro, who helped create the menu and recipe sections of this book and spent untold hours listening to me while I created the final chapters. Thanks also to my dear friend and associate Karen Jarmon, a marketing expert, who was so patient and steadfast with her ability to ground my enthusiasm and focus. Our high school English teacher from West Hartford, Connecticut, Mr. Harris, would be proud! My gratitude goes out to Kathryn Mays Wright for her creative and technical assistance.

My professional and most esteemed colleagues and friends—Nan Fuchs, PhD; Steve Sinatra, MD; Julian Whitaker, MD; Fred Pescatore, MD; Rich Delany, MD; Bruce Blinzler, ND; Kenneth Piller, ND; Paul Schutz, DC; Brad Reed, DC; Noel Baker, DC; Jay Erickson, DC; Michael and Jo Len Schoor; Vicki Accardi; John and Susan Carlson; Sue Swenson; Frankie Boyer; Judy Williams; Kay Channell; Lyle Hurd; Roon Frost; Carol Keppler; Carol Brooks; Maggie Jacqua; Jenny Thompson; Melissa Hickle; Rev. Roberta Herzog; Roy Speiser, PhD, DC; Diane Romeo, DC; Jonny Bouden, Phd; Mary Shomon; Melissa McNew, DC; Hal Huggins, DDS; Stuart Nunnally, DDS; Dr. Pat Boone; Larry Breazeal, OD; Don Tyson; Barbara Kinder; Ellen and Dr. Frantz; Karolyn Gazella; Martie Whittekin; Ezra Zeigler; Kathie Moe; Barbara Lee; Chee Chee Philips; Joan Lanning; Jayne Belancio, Liz Beck; Marlena Spray; and Robin Mize—were nurturing in many profound ways to my body, mind, and spirit throughout the creative process.

My most sincere thanks to my loving and devoted Internet community moderators: Janine Forbes, Linda Shapiro, Cathy Gorbenko, Michelle O'Reardon, Nina Moreau, Sue Durand, Charli Sorenson, Carol Ackerman, and Terri White. These women are extraordinary "women of valor." How fortunate I have been to be surrounded by such generous souls.

My deepest love and appreciation go out to my beloved mother and father, Edith and Arthur, who are my unconditional cheerleaders. And, on the home front, I would be remiss if I didn't recognize my personal assistant and home manager, Tami Oliver, for her extraordinary work ethic and meticulous care of my home (and me). Thank you, Jan Cramer, for all you have done on my behalf with such a willing heart.

Finally, all of this has been worthwhile because of James. Forever is *still* as far as I'll go! I love you so...

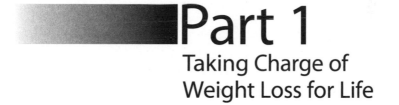

Part 1
Taking Charge of
Weight Loss for Life

1 REVISITING FAT FLUSH

If one advances confidently in the direction of his dreams and endeavors to live the life which he has imagined, he will meet with a success unexpected in common hours.

—Henry David Thoreau

EVERYBODY NEEDS *FAT FLUSH FOR LIFE.*

Plain and simple. Worldwide obesity is on the rise while seven out of ten Americans are overweight or obese. In today's petrochemical world, the fatter you are, the more toxins you are retaining, which is why a detox program should always accompany weight loss. Nearly 100,000 harmful toxins assault your body on a daily basis. Many of these, such as plastics and pesticides, may play a role in obesity by disrupting our metabolism and making us fat. In the weight-loss battle, those of us who support our liver and colon have an enormous advantage because these organs are crucial in ridding our body of fattening chemicals.

These are just some of the reasons why I created Fat Flush, a comprehensive program that combines dieting with detox at the heart of the plan. It has helped people from all ages and stages of life to boost metabolism, transform their body, and keep the weight off for good. I first introduced the concept of Fat Flushing in my very first book, *Beyond Pritikin*, which was published in 1988. Since then, this evolving "diet and detox" has been helping men and women throughout the world safely detoxify as they obtain and maintain their weight-loss goals and improve their health and wellness year round.

Fat Flushing has always been about weight loss, cleansing, and purification. As the name implies, it is designed to literally purge the fats and toxin-laden fluids from your body. But people tell me that it delivers so much more. Fat Flushing gives them a new way of thinking about their overall well-being because, when they begin to Fat Flush, so many "symptoms" of poor health start to disappear. In fact, the unique detox part of the program ultimately leads to benefits such as glowing skin, a dramatic reduction in the appearance of cellulite, high energy levels, more clarity, balanced blood chemistry and hormones, and improved overall health and wellness. It's no wonder Fat Flushing has become synonymous with looking and feeling younger.

THE FAT FLUSHING PHENOMENON

Imitation is the most sincere form of flattery. Fat Flush has been the basic template and motivation behind a myriad of other diets, cleanses, juicing fasts, and detox regimens out there. But not one of these copycats gets the stellar results year in and year out that the Fat Flush program can claim—for reasons I will explain in just a moment.

The concept of Fat Flushing has revolutionized weight loss and changed the way Americans diet by introducing the principle of detox dieting. Over the past two decades millions of men and women have used the basic cleansing protocol. In fact, a 2009 *New York Times* article[1] serves as a testament to the evergreen and enduring popularity of Fat Flushing. The article highlighted the increasingly popular detox craze by featuring a successful Fat Flusher, forty-eight-year-old businessman Randall Hansen, PhD. After losing over seventy pounds using *The Fat Flush Plan*, Dr. Hansen still continued to do an annual Fat Flush cleanse (losing an average of ten pounds in two weeks) to maintain health and weight.

The article also pointed out that almost all of the nearly fifteen thousand spas nationwide now offer some type of detox treatment. In 2008, new food and drink products listing "detox" on the label increased by nearly 500 percent (up to 54 percent from only 15 percent in 2003). It appears that detoxing is here to stay. And Fat Flush still leads the pack.

WHY IT'S TIME FOR FAT FLUSH FOR LIFE

As I traveled throughout the country, appearing on TV and on radio promoting Fat Flush, I took questions from thousands of my followers. Some expressed concern that the Fat Flush food choices were too limited for "real life," while others had severe time constraints when it came to planning, shopping, and cooking meals. There were also those who were frustrated, feeling their diet programs required cooking meals separately from the rest of the family. I learned some even turned down party invitations, feeling they would "pig out" and sabotage their progress by making off-plan food and alcohol choices.

To achieve long-term weight-loss success for everybody, I knew I needed to develop practical new options that were less stringent and "more relaxed" for real people. With the benefit of new scientific breakthroughs and product discoveries, I realized it was time for a broader program—*Fat Flush for Life*.

This book will help you achieve even more dramatic and sustained results using a simplified, flexible, and timesaving program based upon the latest fat-busting science. I have listened to Fat Flushers' feedback and have created Fat Flush for

Life to be ideal for newcomers with busy schedules and large amounts of weight to lose as well as program veterans who are ready to kick up their metabolism another notch or two.

What really sets this book apart is its year-round approach. For each season of the year, I've provided a Fat Flush plan that integrates the detoxifying principles of the diet with a corresponding workout and wellness program. You will learn how to take advantage of your body and mind's response to the seasons to reap the greatest Fat Flushing benefits.

Among other unique diet features in this book, you'll be Fat Flushing with an ancient superseed that has made a modern-day comeback, a green superfood drink that is a perfect complement to more comprehensive cleansing, and a powdered probiotic that doubles as a sweetener. There are many more added attractions in the diet, fitness, and wellness arenas that represent significant superdetox advances. Here are more specifics of what you'll find:

New Foods and Supplements
- Chia seeds, the staple food of the Aztecs, Mayans, and Native Americans because of their high omega-3, fiber, and rich, plant-based calcium content
- Green Life Cocktail, rich in cleansing and healing chlorophyll, which helps oxygenate and purify the system
- A probiotic sweetener to increase beneficial gut bacteria and optimize weight loss
- Fish oil as an alternative to flaxseed oil because it reduces tummy fat
- Iodine-rich sea veggies and seasoning that help normalize thyroid function to increase metabolism

New Fat Flushes
- Winter, Spring, Summer, and Autumn Fat Flushing approaches
- A vegetarian plan for Autumn Fat Flush that features plant proteins, which reset metabolism
- A 5-Day Hot Metabolism Booster to break diet plateaus

New Meal Plans and Recipes
- Copper-controlling meal plans that address the surprising connection between copper overload and slow metabolism
- A 7-day full-week sample menu for the Pre–Fat Flush week
- Feasts and festivities menus designed for celebrations and holidays yearlong
- Easy, time-saving, and budget-friendly recipes
- Fat Flush on the Fly recommendations for "legal" convenience foods on the menus

New Options
- Seasonal wellness guides that highlight advanced detox techniques, including the age-old technique of oil pulling, a form of oral cleansing that heals and detoxifies the entire body
- Seasonal fitness plans tailored to the weight-loss and detoxification aspects of the program

FAT FLUSHING: WHY IT WORKS

Although others have eagerly jumped on the Fat Flush bandwagon and tried to repackage the Fat Flushing concept, most other detox diets are totally missing out on the two most crucial aspects of cleansing: the liver and the lymphatic system.

With a whole new breed of toxins threatening health, the need for detox has never been greater. Think estrogen "mimics" in preservatives and pesticides; perchlorate (a derivative of rocket fuel), antibiotics, and drugs in our water supply; electromagnetic energy fields (EMFs) from cell phones and other Wi-Fi sources; and phthalates (a new variety of plastics), for starters. But can our liver and lymph handle it?

The Grand Central Stations of your body's detox functions, the liver and the lymphatic system are ignored, overlooked, or completely misunderstood by most so-called detox experts and by Western medicine as a whole. The fact is that "unprepared" cleansing in today's toxic world can make you really, really sick if you don't pay attention to these major detoxifying systems.

In a nutshell, Fat Flushing takes into account some surprising links between weight loss and your liver, lymphatic system, omega fats, stress, insulin, and "false fat."

Here are the six core Fat Flush commandments:

1. Love Your Liver

Fat Flush is dedicated first and foremost to supporting the liver in its daunting role as the body's purifier.

In reality, the liver is perfectly designed to detoxify itself automatically, without any help from you or Fat Flush, for that matter. As the body's premier detoxifier (think of it as the filter in your personal engine) and fat-burning organ, the liver has an amazing built-in process that is in charge of breaking down *everything* that comes its way, from chemicals, preservatives, and heavy metals to the food and beverages you ingest.

Ah, but here's the rub.

For the detox process to work smoothly, your body needs a plethora of heavy-duty, nutritional elements to keep the detox pathways working optimally and to break down toxins. So, you need to be *very* well nourished to detox.

A liver clogged with poisons or excess fats cannot perform its fat-burning and other essential duties, including maintaining blood sugar levels, storing glycogen, synthesizing and normalizing blood proteins, and helping to keep your body in hormonal balance. A poorly functioning liver results in stagnation. Freeing up your liver to do its job may be the single most important step you ever take in improving your overall health and achieving your weight-loss goals permanently.

The Fat Flush program accomplishes this task in several ways. One is through the antioxidant/phenol-rich cranberry and water mixture you will be drinking during each seasonal Fat Flush to keep those detox pathways moving right along. And the benefits of cranberries keep on accruing. Cranberries were analyzed with other fruits for their antioxidant power by measuring their ORAC value (oxygen radical absorbance capacity). Cranberries register a 9,584 ORAC value, compared to the second runner-up (raspberries), which were only 4,882.[2] So cranberries are powerful medicine in neutralizing harmful free radicals and preventing them from taking a foothold in the body.

Daily intake of foods in the liver-loving veggie cruciferous family (think cauliflower, cabbage, broccoli, and Brussels sprouts) also speeds the breakdown of fat-storing toxins and keeps new body fat from forming. Lemon and water first thing in the morning helps to thin out bile and tone up both the kidneys and liver. Eggs (preferably from chickens that don't do drugs) are part of the regimen because their high sulfur content and lecithin helps the liver's detox pathways and aids in the forming of bile salts.

Fat Flush also includes several servings of whey protein to provide amino acid building blocks that are precursors to glutathione—the liver's premier antioxidant, which destroys free radicals and detoxifies carcinogens and all kinds of poisons in the body.

When you clean up your act, the liver and its beautiful bile are nourished with the right foods and supplements, which will ensure efficient fat metabolism as well as efficient elimination of toxins and wastes.

2. Love Your Lymph

If the liver is your body's filter, then the lymph channels are your body's drainage system. Your lymphatic system is the foundation of your immune system and includes your spleen, tonsils, and thymus. If you have never heard of the lymphatic system, you are not alone. So many people, even those into detox, have no idea about the crucial role this system plays in health and in weight loss.

The lymphatic system is a complex network of needle-thin tubes filled with fluid that continually bathes our cells and then carries away the body's "garbage"—toxins, waste products of metabolism, fat globules, and excess liquid—to filters called lymph nodes, where these substances are stored and then neutralized. But whereas blood has a pump (your heart) to keep it moving, the lymph must be pumped by the movement of muscles or through deep breathing. (You can begin to see how a sedentary lifestyle can affect your health.)

The lymph, like the liver, can be overloaded with chemicals, pesticides, and a variety of pollutants that can shut down lymphatic flow. Plus, the everyday stress we are under also is a lymph stressor. The muscles and motion of breathing are a primary way to move lymph and when we're under stress, our breathing becomes shallower.

So what does this mean for your waistline? First off, if your lymph isn't flowing, your tissues aren't draining excess fluid. This creates a backlog that results in bloating. Waterlogged tissues can cause your body to swell up to two sizes—weighing in with an extra ten to fifteen pounds—yikes! A lazy lymphatic system may also be connected to cellulite because backed-up fluid "sticks" to fat cells. Last but not least, waterlogged tissues interfere with nutrient and oxygen absorption and utilization, so cell starvation starts to take place.

The *Fat Flush for Life* program cleanses your lymph with a special fitness regimen that focuses on rebounding—the best exercise for the lymphatics due to the gentle bouncing action. The exercise component is fortified with Fat Flushing Superstar Foods that saturate the system with detoxifying enzymes, antioxidants, and phytonutrients. The Cranberry H_2O drink in the program, for example, is packed with flavonoids, enzymes, and organic acids that appear to act like natural digestive enzymes. From my observations, cranberry helps to digest lumpy deposits of lymphatic waste, which could be one of the key reasons Fat Flushers report that their cellulite disappears.

People who detox their livers and get their lymph flowing also notice they have clear, smooth, glowing skin and a toned body. Sugar cravings vanish. More nutrients get to the cells and more calories become energy when lymph flows freely. Swelling and bloating are a thing of the past; radiant good health takes their place. So, healing the lymphatics is a big deal, not only for Fat Flushing but also for disease control. Those of you with Crohn's disease, please take note. In the January 2008 issue of the journal *Gut*, it was reported that Crohn's is caused by inflammation and thickening of the lymphatics connected to the intestines—not by an autoimmune disease or a genetic condition, as previously thought.[3][4]

3. Eat the Right Fat to Lose Fat

GLA and Brown Fat. A flurry of new studies about fighting fat with fat came out in the *New England Journal of Medicine* in early 2009. The media heralded these studies as the newest obesity theory, claiming that good fat, also known as brown fat because of its color, is a potent regulator of metabolism and weight. The research said that brown fat is deficient in overweight people and is primarily activated by cold.[5] [6]

This good fat, which triggers the body to burn more calories and generate more body heat, is key in keeping infants warm. By adulthood, brown fat is metabolically inactive in many individuals. However—what the researchers completely overlooked is the role of the essential fatty acid, gamma linolenic acid, more commonly known as GLA. Since the 1980s, it has been known that GLA stimulates brown fat activity through its prostaglandin pathways.[7] [8] This is exactly why GLA has played a crucial role in Fat Flush since the origins of the program. It is found in its most balanced form in black currant seed oil, although borage and evening primrose oil are other rich sources.[9] GLA is also included in the starter Fat Flush Kit as the GLA-90s supplement.

Omega-3s and Omega-6s. Fats high in the omega-3s (such as chia seeds, flaxseed oil, and fish oil) and the omega-6s (GLA and conjugated linoleic acid, or CLA), are all crucial to weight loss and are part of the Fat Flush prescription. Although only GLA mobilizes the metabolically active brown fat, they all reduce inflammation that can trigger weight gain and have the added benefit of helping your body burn off fat more effectively. The omega-3s balance blood sugar, which takes the lid off of cravings while helping to stimulate the production of leptin, an appetite-regulating hormone in fat cells.

In addition, since the omega-3s and omega-6s are polyunsaturated fats, their biochemical structure easily permeates cellular walls, producing satiety and inhibiting overeating, among many other health benefits. Moreover, the essential omegas are necessary for balanced brain function and provide real help for such problems as attention-deficit/hyperactivity disorder (ADHD). They prevent blood clotting, repair tissue damage caused by clogged arteries, lower triglycerides and high blood pressure, and protect the body from autoimmune disease, such as rheumatoid arthritis.

CLA, known as a "critical" omega-6 fatty acid, is produced by grazing animals (e.g., cows) from the linoleic acid in the grass they eat. Taken as a concentrated dietary supplement, it prompts the body to burn stored fat as energy, resulting in a decrease in overall body fat and a proportional increase in lean muscle tissue, which in turn burns even more calories. Like the omega-3s, CLA also helps balance blood sugar levels.[10]

Omega-9s. Fats from the omega-9s (olive oil and macadamia nut oil) are also weight-loss aids. They are high in a particular type of monounsaturated fatty acid, or MUFA, known as oleic acid. This acid keeps *Candida* from reproducing, which keeps yeast from overgrowing and causing bloating and weight gain. In 2007, a small but highly popularized study was published in *Diabetes Care* in which Spanish researchers discovered that a MUFA-high diet contributes to a svelte belly by inhibiting tummy fat accumulation.[11] For lifelong overall health, these oils provide satiety, help lower cholesterol, reduce the risk of heart attack, protect arteries, and support breast health. They are also the best flavor carriers for the anti-inflammatory pharmacy of spices that Fat Flush incorporates, such as ginger, garlic, turmeric, dry mustard, cayenne, oregano, cloves, and cinnamon.

4. Stress Less (and Sleep More) for Less Fat

Cortisol, the stress hormone secreted by the adrenal glands, is a fat-promoting hormone that creates tummy fat, much to our dismay. When you are under any type of stress it triggers enzymes to store more fat, because your body believes there is "danger ahead" and instant energy may be needed. Since deep abdominal fat contains four times more cortisol receptors than do other fat sites, cortisol is drawn to it.

One of the secrets of low-stress success is simply getting the proper amount of sleep. Too little sleep *can* make you fat. A study that tracked the effect of sleep habits on the weight gain of nearly seventy thousand middle-aged women recently confirmed this principle. This research showed that women who slept for five hours per night generally weighed more than women who slept for seven hours per night. In fact, women who only got five versus seven hours of sleep were 32 percent more likely to experience major weight gain (an increase of thirty-three pounds or more). Plus these sleep-deprived women were shown to be 15 percent more likely to become obese over the course of the sixteen-year study.

When it comes to sleep, cortisol can cause a real domino effect on metabolism and overall health. Insufficient sleep can cause the release of cortisol and stimulate hunger. Cortisol surges throughout the night may keep you from sleeping and then impact changes in metabolic rate, leading to a decreased ability to burn fat. As sleep levels decrease, cortisol increases, so elevated cortisol levels are connected with sleep-deprived weight gain.

In fact, a lack of sleep *creates* cravings. Researchers at the University of Chicago who deprived healthy young adults of sleep found that in addition to increased overall appetite, the volunteers experienced a particular surge in cravings for sweet and salty foods.[12]

According to a landmark sleep study in the *Journal of the American Medical Association*, if you sleep between 7.5 and 8.5 hours per night, you will secrete half as much cortisol than those who get 6.5 hours or less. Furthermore, inadequate sleep interferes with the body's ability to metabolize carbohydrates and depresses leptin levels.[13] As readers of my *Fat Flush Plan* are aware, going to sleep by 10:00 p.m. is an essential part of the Fat Flushing lifestyle habits, to ensure quality sleep and enough sleep—the best diet secret of all. The unavoidable action of natural aging compounds this fattening cycle. When we are young our body regulates cortisol levels naturally by creating more cortisol in the morning (two to three times more), allowing us to start our day full of energy, and then our body naturally decreases cortisol levels in the evening so that we can easily fall into the much needed sleep. Unfortunately by middle age our baseline cortisol level naturally begins to rise, making it tougher to go to sleep and to stay asleep. In fact, we become even more sensitive to the additional cortisol created by these same sleep disturbances, triggering even more hormone havoc, accelerating aging and increasing our waistline.

Fat Flush corrects this vicious cycle by limiting cortisol-spiking caffeine in both coffee and tea as well as recommending a meal plan with suitable between-meal snacks to keep cortisol at bay. Journaling is also a stress-controlling, and therefore cortisol-lowering, habit.

Of course, sleeping for at least seven to eight hours is another must. Inadequate sleep also inhibits the body's ability to metabolize carbohydrates, which lead to higher insulin levels, a topic that is addressed next.

5. Lower Your Insulin to Lower Your Weight

Like cortisol, insulin is another fat-promoting hormone. Remember, hormones—and not just calories—dramatically impact weight. Insulin, the key hormone that controls blood sugar levels, is triggered by an excessive intake of carbs. Insulin helps store blood sugar in the liver and tissues as glycogen. However, the body can only store a limited amount of glycogen and any excess is converted to body fat with the assistance of insulin.

Fat-deprived individuals tend to eat too many carbs, programming their insulin levels to remain high. The insulin in turn instructs the body to store fat. So, the key is to keep insulin levels low by eating a diet high in protein and essential fatty acids (all insulin-lowering macronutrients). Eating protein purposely stimulates the pancreas to produce glucagon, the hormone that counteracts insulin and mobilizes fat from storage.

Fat Flush addresses high insulin levels with a balanced diet of lean protein, low-glycemic, slow-burning carbohydrates, omega-3 oils and foods, as well as omega-6 botanical oils. Fat Flush features a wide variety of fruits, vegetables, and "clean carbs" (starchy veggies, cereals, and nongluten grains) that are both low-glycemic and hypoallergenic so they do not create an inflammatory response leading to water retention, adding insult to injury. This is why the most commonly reactive foods—like wheat, milk, sugar, and corn—are eliminated on Fat Flush.

It is also interesting to note that sleep, as we have seen with cortisol, also plays a part in balancing insulin. According to the National Sleep Foundation, sleep loss can lead to insulin resistance and reduced levels of growth hormones that help to regulate fat and muscle proportions.[14]

6. Recognize False Fat

Weight gain can also be related to "false fat"—meaning water-logged tissues, which can result from numerous underlying causes: prescription medicines (over fifty have been connected to weight gain), food sensitivities, hormonal imbalances, and insufficient water and protein consumption. Many medicines, including antidepressants, steroid hormones, and anticonvulsants can cause weight gain by spiking appetite and decreasing metabolism.

When it comes to food sensitivities, research published in *Lancet* and the *New England Journal of Medicine* strongly makes the case that chemicals involved with toxic responses to common foods inhibit the body's ability to burn stored fat. This can lead to food addictions and binging due to the temporary "high" (an opioid-type chemical response) that eating the wrong food can produce.[15] [16]

A whole slew of troubling symptoms are related to food sensitivities, from unexplained mood swings to panic attacks, sinusitis, chronic fatigue, extreme tiredness after eating, a racing pulse, puffy eyes, and swelling beneath the eyes. Weight can yo-yo up and down every day by as much as five to ten pounds due to an inflammatory response whereby the body holds water to dilute the perceived "toxin."

Note that unlike food sensitivities, a true food allergy (such as a peanut allergy) can lead to anaphylactic shock, an allergic response during which the body releases histamines that cause tissues to swell and inhibit breathing. More common allergic responses to food include skin reactions such as hives and eczema. But food sensitivities are not always as immediate as allergic responses; they may have a delayed response that can manifest up to two days after the "toxic" food is ingested, making it difficult to pinpoint the problematic food.

Fat Flush helps you overcome food sensitivities by eliminating the most commonly "reactive" foods—wheat, milk, yeast, and sugar. When these foods are slowly reintroduced back into the program, you are encouraged to note your responses in a food journal so that you can better determine the possible food cause of that bloating, gas, "false fat" weight gain (water retention), and/or stalled weight loss.

Meet a Fat Flusher for Life

Randall H., DeLand, Florida
48 years old; PhD; entrepreneur; 8-year
Fat Flusher; lost 75 pounds

I had reached the heaviest I have ever been—close to 270 pounds—and was wearing 2XL men's shirts—untucked. All my business suits no longer fit me and I refused to wear ties and such because they looked like they were choking me with my double/triple chins. I had kind of given up before Fat Flush came into my life.

Even though I wanted to believe, I had been on enough diets that I was skeptical. The two-week Fat Flush was… an eye-opener. I had horrible headaches the first few days, from caffeine and sugar withdrawal, but once those went away, I started feeling better. At the end of the two weeks, I had lost about 16 pounds.

I moved on to Phase 2, along with adding a daily exercise regimen that combined walking and bicycling. Over the course of the next 6 months, I lost another 65 pounds…dropping to about 188 (which some people told me made me too skinny) and to a size medium shirt! I eventually settled on about 195 as my ideal weight—and maintain that weight today—eight years and going strong. I do the two-week cleanse at least once a year to break some bad habits that creep back in and to knock off a few pounds.

Since the time I started getting annual physicals and blood work, my bad cholesterol numbers have continued to go down, my good cholesterol up, and my ratio is extremely strong. My triglycerides are also very low.

I believe the tenets of Fat Flush—healthy eating, good exercise, positive mental outlook, and daily supplements—have put me in a place today that I never could have imagined before Fat Flush.

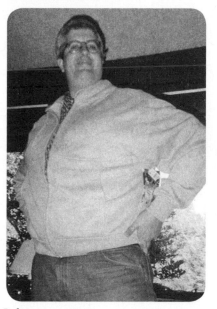

Before

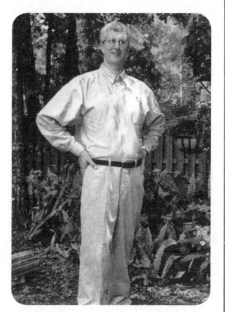

After

When food sensitivities are eliminated, weight loss becomes a no-brainer. Fat Flushers typically say, it's not what they are eating but what they are *not* eating that is making them lose weight without any caloric concerns. In fact, many Fat Flushers eat more food, not less, than ever before.

Fat Flushing helps rid you of "false fat" by supporting the liver's ability to better metabolize all drugs and prescription medications through liver-healing foods. Each stage of the program is packed with cruciferous veggies that provide sulforaphane, a phytonutrient that triggers the liver to produce more detoxifying enzymes; green leafy vegetables high in purifying chlorophyll and magnesium that also have natural diuretic properties; high–vitamin C citrus; and sulfur-rich foods such as garlic, onion, eggs, and daikon radish that also help the liver eliminate toxins. Zinc-rich, high-protein foods (lean beef, eggs, pumpkin seeds) counter a copper buildup in the liver that can also impede its function.

Fat Flush for Life is about moving forward. The next chapter details the revolutionary concepts and cutting-edge science behind this evolving lifelong eating and wellness program. It partners the classic Fat Flush foundation with wellness and fitness for a super seasonal detox program—that is better than ever—for permanent weight loss.

2 REFINING FAT FLUSH

Health is a journey, not a destination.

—Anonymous

FAT FLUSHING HAS always defied conventional wisdom.

Its novel approach to weight loss first made waves in *The Fat Flush Plan*, when I suggested there are "hidden" factors, beyond the control of diet, exercise, and your own willpower, that are making you fat. Research now confirms that weight loss is also about an array of newly uncovered concerns that are contributing to the obesity epidemic. When you address and correct seemingly unrelated factors such as your body's microbes, omega-3 and iodine deficiency, and copper overload, you can drop those pounds for good. You'll restore your body's natural ability to regulate metabolism and detoxify. Controlling what is really weighing you down might just change your total outlook as well as your outfit.

So let's take a more careful look at the new scientific research that has enhanced many of the fundamental Fat Flush protocols.

GUT BACTERIA TIED TO WEIGHT LOSS

Taking supplemental probiotics (beneficial bacteria or friendly flora) may be the real deal when it comes to losing weight. Fat Flushing now includes a probiotic, Flora-Key, which can also be used as a natural sweetener, in response to new findings suggesting a strong connection between obesity and the levels of certain types of bacteria in the gut. In a study published in *Nature* (December 2006), the researchers basically found that without the right amounts of friendly bacteria, animals got "twice as fat" and utilized more calories from the same amount of food than those with the more normal bacteria ratio.[1]

For years, beneficial bacteria (or friendly flora) have been well known to fight yeast, combat disease-causing bacteria, help clean out parasites, and break down toxins in the body. Conversely, a lack of the beneficial bacteria have been connected to many health problems, including ulcers, irritable bowel syndrome (IBS), chronic fatigue, eczema and psoriasis, asthma, and more. And now there is a connection to weight.

Probiotic means "for life." Probiotics play an important role in the digestion of foods and help to produce B vitamins, vitamin K, as well as digesting fiber—the short-chain fatty acids upon which your colon desperately relies. In the right balance of power, a ratio of 85 to 15 in favor of the "good guy" bacteria, probiotics are so vital to good health that they are considered an "organ" by many experts. In reality, these friendly flora also make up most of your immune system, because 60 percent of your immune system's receptor cells are in your large intestine and another 15 percent reside in the small intestine.

Probiotics represent the next wave of health and healing and are intimately involved with every organ, tissue, and health concern of the body. It should come as no surprise that researchers made a link between weight and gut bacteria in two studies published in *Nature*.[2] [3]

This groundbreaking research, conducted at Washington University's Center for Genome Sciences, initiated a whole science called "infectobesity" that looks at obesity from the microbial and viral standpoint. Simply put: viruses and bacteria may impact the absorption of food and influence gut hormones that regulate appetite and metabolic rate.

For years, probiotics have been an integral part of my dietary protocols in such books as *The Fast Track Detox Diet* and *The Gut Flush Plan*. For the basic weight loss and cleansing purposes of *Fat Flush for Life*, I am recommending a powdered probiotic supplement that I have been using in private practice for over a decade, Flora-Key. It can do double duty as an immune booster and natural sweetener because we are cutting out sugar, sugar alcohols, and even artificial sweeteners such as aspartame or Splenda. (My one exception is the "legal cheat" stevia.)

In *Fat Flush for Life*, Flora-Key is a key dietary ingredient in no-heat foods such as frappés, fruits, and the Green Life Cocktail superfood drink. It contains a basic combination of lactobacillus, bifidobacterium, and frucooligosaccharides (FOS) from complex sugars that function as a prebiotic. A prebiotic is a food that feeds the beneficial bacteria while discouraging pathogens. FOS is a naturally occurring sweetener in fruits and some vegetables. It tastes sweet but the molecules are too big to be digested by the body as sugar, so it doesn't affect blood sugar levels. It also can't be utilized by *Candida* and other yeasts. The best news about FOS, though, is that it provides a benefit that none of the other sweeteners do: It nourishes and promotes the growth of friendly intestinal bacteria such as bifidobacteria in your large intestine without feeding pathogenic bacteria.

This makes it a potentially good-for-you sweetener for people struggling with weight, yeast infections, and other gastrointestinal (GI) disorders. With Flora-Key, you get the best of both worlds: a probiotic fed by a prebiotic. You can take two to three teaspoons per day.

For heavy-duty immune enhancement, I stand by Dr. Ohhira's Probiotic 12 Plus, found in health food stores all over the country. It contains all the beneficial lactic acid bacteria found in humans. Perhaps its major claim to fame is its patented TH10 strain that neutralizes the "smartbugs" (such as salmonella and *E. coli*) that spread food-borne disease and are resistant to antibiotics. More than a probiotic, this product represents a flora-balancing system. It improves gut pH for the benefit of other friendly flora while requiring no refrigeration and is dairy, soy, and gluten free. Best of all, the product is backed by nearly fifteen years of university-backed scientific research.

FISH OILS LINKED TO TUMMY FAT

Gaining an awareness of bad and good fats is critical to maintaining health and achieving weight goals. Along with high-lignan flaxseed oil, fish oil is another "good fat" option. Reams of research demonstrate how fish oil can make you thinner, soothe arthritis, improve focus, protect the eyes, lower cholesterol, balance blood sugar, prevent heart disease, and boost brainpower.

In terms of weight loss alone, in another study published in the *American Journal of Clinical Nutrition*, individuals who consumed fish oil and walked for forty-five minutes three times a week lost up to five more pounds than the control group! Researchers noted that the combination of fish oil and exercise significantly reduced body fat, which indicates the potential benefit of a combined treatment strategy for optimizing body composition in overweight or obese subjects.[4] *Fat Flush for Life* reflects this research with the addition of a fish oil option to the original protocol.

IODINE DEFICIENCY AND HYPOTHYROIDISM

Hypothyroidism (underactivity of the thyroid gland, your body's energy burner and thermostat) is epidemic. Next to diabetes, hypothyroidism is the most common endocrine disorder in the country these days. I hear from women of all ages, starting in their late twenties, how the doctor has put them on thyroid meds such as Synthyroid and Armour. Although the latest statistics suggest that four out of ten Americans have hypothyroidism, I think the number may even be higher due to subclinical thyroid conditions.

A low-functioning thyroid will slow down your body's metabolism as well as reduce your heart and muscle strength. Besides the inability to lose weight, hypothyroidism is linked to depression, hair loss, poor eyebrow growth (especially the outer third of the brow), dry skin, irritability, aching wrists, fluid retention, constipation, a coarse voice, decreased blood pressure, and premature graying of the hair.

The connection between thyroid function and iodine levels became clear about sixty years ago. The thyroid gland depends upon iodine to make its hormones.

Why is this important? One of these thyroid hormones, thyroxin (T4), *regulates energy metabolism*, meaning *it determines how fast your body burns food for energy.* The bottom line is that iodine is able to restore balance to thyroid hormones whether they are high or low.

According to David Brownstein, MD, over the past three decades, our iodine intake decreased 50 percent while thyroid disorders (hypothyroidism, auto-immune thyroid disorders, and thyroid cancer) increased significantly. Dr. Brownstein tested more than one thousand people at his Michigan clinic and discovered that 95 percent had low, inadequate iodine levels. His findings mirror results found by a national laboratory that tested more than four thousand individuals.[5]

How can you tell if your thyroid level is low? Other than the symptoms I describe above, the best way to know for sure is to be tested. You can test and effectively treat your iodine levels by doing a special, iodine-loading test pioneered by the visionary endocrinologist Guy Abraham, MD. (See resources, page 257.) Dr. Abraham's 24-hour urine test found that most individuals need about 50 mg of iodine per day—far more than the recommended daily allowance (RDA) of 150 mcgs.[6]

As my friend and colleague Nan Fuchs, PhD, points out, although 150 mcg of iodine per day is adequate, there are many benefits to taking more—*especially for women.*[7] In higher amounts, iodine acts as an adaptogen, a substance that increases the body's ability to adapt to stress, and plays a significant role in preventing such disorders as polycystic ovary disease, fibrocystic breast disease, sleep apnea, diabetes, cardiac arrhythmia, hypertension, and hormone imbalances. Since women have larger breasts than men and iodine is concentrated in the breast tissue, women simply need more iodine to protect against disease and possibly cancer.

It is important to also note that a low hydrochloric acid level (HCL), healthy stomach acid, can be triggered by an iodine insufficiency because we need iodine to enable chloride to enter the stomach cells. Without enough HCL, the body won't digest protein or use iron or calcium and magnesium. As we hit the age of sixty, our HCL decreases by almost half. Increasing your iodine is one good way to increase HCL production naturally, thereby improving digestion.

In light of the importance of iodine to so many bodily functions, you will be shoring up your iodine levels with iodine-rich sea vegetables (hijiki, wakame, kombu, agar, and nori) at least twice a week on the *Fat Flush for Life* menu plans and incorporating an iodine-rich seasoning (Seaweed Gomasio) for flavor and health.

COPPER OVERLOAD AND HYPOTHYROIDISM

Besides being affected by iodine, your thyroid can be suppressed by an elevated copper level. Copper, like iodine, can also inhibit the conversion of the thyroid hormone thyroxin, resulting in a slowdown of metabolism. In my experience with tissue mineral analysis (TMA) over the past two decades, I have observed that an elevated tissue level of copper is frequently linked with hypothyroidism, especially when the zinc-to-copper ratio is higher than ten to one (ideal is eight to one in favor of zinc). In fact, women with low zinc levels also tend to have high copper, a connection that I've found in 70 to 80 percent of women. Zinc is typically very deficient in vegetarians, individuals under stress, and those who don't eat zinc-rich sources of foods such as red meat, eggs, and pumpkin seeds.

A copper-zinc imbalance also affects the liver's ability to detoxify. Copper and zinc are both needed to activate key liver enzymes; if they are out of balance, your liver is out of balance. This leaves the liver less able to eliminate toxins, including excess copper. The result is a cycle of high copper and poor liver function.

Copper levels seem to rise and fall in tandem with estrogen levels. If you are deficient in zinc, the balancing mineral to copper, and/or lacking in progesterone, the hormone that balances estrogen, copper levels tend to rise. Weight gain as well as frontal headaches, menstrual irregularities, food cravings, mood swings, fatigue, depression, and yeast infections are all common symptoms of copper overload.

Lowered adrenal gland activity is another key culprit behind high copper levels. Interestingly, TMA test results from my clinical experience show that seven out of ten women have weak adrenal glands. Adrenal gland activity is required to stimulate the liver's production of ceruloplasmin, the leading copper-binding protein. With diminished adrenal activity, unbound copper starts to gather in various tissues, organs, and glands—such as the thyroid.

Selected Foods with a High Copper Content, in milligrams per 100 grams:

Yeast, dried	4.98	Sesame seeds	1.59
Regular tea, bag	4.80	Brazil nuts	1.53
Cocoa powder	3.87	Coffee (ground)	1.26
Chocolate (bitter)	2.67	Soybeans	1.17
Wheat germ	2.39	Curry powder	1.07
Sunflower seeds	1.77		

Meet a Fat Flusher for Life

Michelle O., Atlanta, Georgia
54 years old; educator; 4-year Fat Flusher;
lost more than 50 pounds

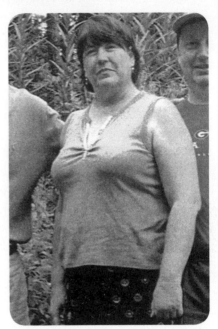

Before

My life changed on Saturday, August 20, 2005. That was the day I bought Ann Louise Gittleman's *Fast Track Detox Diet*. And since that day the quality of my life has increased so dramatically, that if it hadn't happened to me, I would have a hard time believing it was possible. Once I completed *Fast Track*, I started on Fat Flush, and I've been "flushing" ever since.

I lost over 50 pounds and went from wearing a size 20 to wearing a size 8—with the occasional size 6 thrown in for good measure.

You might be wondering what my life was like before I began following [the Fat Flush] protocols. Well, in a word—unhealthy. I was at my highest weight ever; I had aching joints and low, low, low energy. I was close to resigning myself to being overweight and unhealthy for the remainder of my life, which to be honest, I was afraid wouldn't be a very long one.

With my commitment to following these plans, I found energy levels I didn't think were possible, health that is greater than I have had in my entire life, a more toned and shapely body than I had in years. And my enthusiasm for life burst into full bloom. Along with those marvelous benefits came compliments from friends, family, and co-workers. And I have to admit, I never get tired of hearing people say, "Michelle, you look great!"

Being part of the [online] Forum over the past two and a half years has given me an incredible amount of support. Knowing that I was part of an international group of people who were dedicated to reclaiming their health was an inspiration and an incentive to do my best. I'd say the Forum was one of the key factors of my success. Would I ever go back to my life before Fast Track and Fat Flush? Not for 50 million dollars. This is the life I was meant to have. This is the level of health I want, and this is the way I'm going to live the rest of my life.

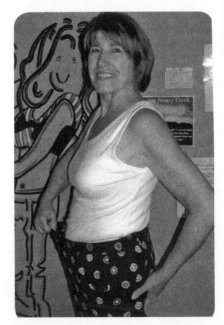

After

There are many external sources for copper exposure. Copper occurs naturally in drinking water in some areas and in others it is actually added to municipal water sources as copper sulfate. Copper water pipes, copper cookware, birth control pills, copper IUDs, dental fillings, and crowns—all put you at risk for copper overload. But the interesting thing is that the typical vegetarian menu contains a high-copper and low-zinc assortment of foods. Add to this a diet high in phytate-rich grains (such as whole grains) known to lower zinc levels, and the trouble becomes twofold.

The truth is we need only a pinch of copper in our bodies. The average person ingests 2.5 to 5.0 milligrams of copper per day; those who eat a vegetarian diet typically take in more. The range that is considered safe and adequate to meet our needs is 1.5 to 3.0 milligrams per day; the recommended dietary intake for adults is 2.0. In light of the copper overload from the environment, controlling dietary copper is paramount.

In all of the seasonal Fat Flushing menus, including the vegetarian autumn menu, I've made sure to correct the copper-zinc imbalance by cutting down on copper-rich foods (such as chocolate and soy) and including more zinc. The following box will give you a better idea of dietary copper culprits.

As you can see, *Fat Flush for Life* takes its inspiration from the latest fat-busting science, my professional experience, and my heartfelt desire to make the program more well rounded and convenient for those on a workaday schedule. As you read through this book, you will discover that *Fat Flush for Life* will retrain your taste buds, resculpt your body, and restore your immunity with a year-round, self-care approach that addresses your spirit, too.

3 UNDERSTANDING THE SEASONAL FAT FLUSH APPROACH

I MENTIONED EARLIER that what makes *Fat Flush for Life* unique is its year-round approach. The influence of the seasons on the delicate balance of your body is one of the most vital but overlooked aspects of total health. The seasons, which last approximately three months each, have their own rhythm and character, bringing with them temperature and weather changes as well as different lengths of daylight, all of which affect your health. Amazingly, this is true even for those who live in geographical areas where the seasons are less apparent, such as Florida, where it's warm most of the time, or Alaska, where it's cold. Our body responds to the changing of the seasons regardless of climate.

Fat Flush for Life is designed to help you tap into nature's harmonious cycles by using special foods, teas, herbs, wellness techniques, and indoor and outdoor fitness workouts to keep your body cool in spring and summer and heated up in autumn and winter. Based upon the principles of traditional Chinese medicine, this book provides healing strategies for you that will fortify and nurture the major detoxifying organs of the body. The Chinese for centuries have believed that certain organs are activated at particular times of the year and need more tender loving care (TLC):

Winter—kidneys and adrenals **Spring**—liver and gallbladder
Summer—heart and small intestine **Autumn**—lungs and large intestine

Each aspect of this total health plan—diet, fitness, and wellness—is broken down by the four seasons and provides support and nourishment for the corresponding activated organs. The body thrives and metabolism is sparked when we make shifts and changes to our diet, so I've designed a program where you will be in a different stage of Fat Flush for every month of the year. Winter, for example, is the time during which your body slows down and works to conserve energy. A diet featuring denser, warming foods is necessary to replenish and renew your overstressed kidneys and adrenals. Spring, on the other hand, is the time to begin a lighter diet after a winter time of eating fattier, heavier foods. It's the time to get outside once again and allow your body to release those toxic wastes that have been building up after a sedentary winter. The fresh, seasonal springtime produce you'll be eating will counter the excess fat and mucus buildup from winter and help refresh your liver and gallbladder.

The dietary recommendations feature seasonal suggestions for foods that are not just "in season," but are truly supportive of the associated organ and the challenges of the weather. For example, summer is the time to turn careful attention to your heart. Potassium-rich tomatoes, along with cooling salads and abundant salad vegetables, especially jicama and cucumbers, are an ideal way to balance summertime heat.

The heavy-duty detox that begins Summer Fat Flush is best completed during warmer weather for the simple reason that cold acts as a stressor to the system. Cold makes the body contract and thereby impedes the flow of toxic wastes. Heat, on the other hand, is relaxing, allowing for more effortless elimination.

HOW TO USE THIS BOOK

Before we jump into the seasonal Fat Flushing plans, part 1 ends with a rundown of the signature Fat Flush diet staples and strategies that offer the most therapeutic properties for cleansing and weight loss. These abundant superfoods and supplements offer the highest level of nutrition—phytonutrients, antioxidants, omega-3s, chlorophyll, soluble fiber, probiotics, amino acids, and the time-tested Fat Flush Kit. You'll also learn about the legendary Parcells' Clorox Bath that helps remove pesticides and more from your fresh foods so you don't always have to buy organic.

At this point, you'll be ready to begin part 2, the Pre–Fat Flush Diet, a seven-day meal plan that sets the stage and prepares you for full-fledged Fat Flushing. You should start with the Pre–Fat Flush Diet regardless of which season you begin *Fat Flush for Life*.

Part 3, Winter Fat Flush, features choice hypoallergenic (or "clean") carbs as well as thyroid-nourishing sea veggies and probiotics. These will keep you feeling warm and satisfied through the cold winter months while revving up your metabolism and protecting your immunity.

Part 4, Spring Fat Flush, transitions you into a lighter way of eating that takes advantage of fresh, seasonal produce that is critical to the cleansing process and liver support at this time.

Part 5, Summer Fat Flush, marks the beginning of the accelerated detox. It continues to focus on nourishing the liver and the thyroid while releasing accumulated toxins from the lymphatic system and from your stores of fat. Most individuals lose weight extremely quickly during this phase. Once you're done, you'll switch to a more relaxed way of eating until the summer comes to an end.

Part 6, Autumn Fat Flush, unveils the long-anticipated vegetarian Fat Flush diet in which you will be enticed by delicious plant proteins that will fill you up and help to reset your metabolism. A new Fat Flush body protein powder, free of dairy, soy, and gluten (ideal for vegans) is on the menu. Even the hardest core meat-eaters will have no beef with these vegetarian menu plans. This lighter way of eating, similar to Summer Fat Flush, continues to lend itself to optimum cleansing but also gently transitions you into more substantial foods for the onset of colder weather in preparation for winter.

I've also included a 5-Day Hot Metabolism Booster, which will help you break out of diet slumps. This five-day plan makes use of many Fat Flushing favorites and introduces a special cocktail to fire up your metabolism if you hit a weight-loss plateau. You can use the 5-Day Hot Metabolism Booster during any season, whenever you feel you need a little dietary jump start.

Each seasonal Fat Flush is accompanied by a 14-day meal plan that carefully outlines what you should eat morning, noon, and night and between meals. These plans are really just templates that you can use as examples for your own creative menu planning. Many people get hung up thinking they have to follow every sample breakfast, lunch, dinner, and snack to the letter. Not so.

At the beginning of every meal plan in each season, you will find a Fat Flushing Superstar Foods list that allows you to personalize the meal plans to your own tastes. To prevent portion distortion, each category also gives you the serving sizes of each food in that particular food group. By the time you have flushed your way through the entire program, you will have nourished your overworked liver, unclogged your lymph, stoked your thyroid, and overcome food cravings while obtaining and stabilizing your desired weight for life.

Part 6, Fat Flush for Life Menus and Recipes, illustrates just how easy and appealing Fat Flush dining can be. Chapter 20 presents selected menus for feasts and festivities throughout the year when company is coming and you want to show off. Whether it's a Summer Breeze Luncheon that features Chickpea Tahini Pâté and Summer Fruit Crumble, or a Thanksgiving Buffet that delights with Roasted Pumpkin with Cranberries and Quinoa Risotto, these menus will help make your special occasions elegant and wholesome.

Chapter 21 features the complete collection of Fat Flush for Life Recipes with more than seventy-five soon-to-be favorites. You'll especially like the homemade recipes created by veteran Fat Flushers who contributed family favorites like Can't Resist Chick'n Spinach Chili, Sweetie Po' Puffs, and Curried Delicata Squash Bisque to this section. There are many more family and kid-friendly recipes as well as more elaborate dishes for feasts and festivities—all with the Fat Flush seal of approval and tested in our official Fat Flush Kitchens.

SEASONAL WELLNESS

The Fat Flush seasonal diets are only the first piece of this holistic approach to good health. Each season also includes a wellness section that teaches the most effective ways to calm your emotions, to more thoroughly stimulate liver, lymph, and colon cleansing, and to assess underlying nutritional imbalances impacting your overall health. You will be introduced to the best time of the year that your body can benefit from castor oil packs, dry skin brushing, coffee enemas, and colonics. You will also learn about new self-care rituals and ways to pamper yourself with mini-indulgences.

Meet a Fat Flusher for Life

Nikki T., Post Falls, Idaho
34 years old; active working mother; 3-year Fat Flusher; lost 75 pounds

Fat Flush has been life changing. I have completely transformed from who I used to be to a younger, more vibrant and skinnier, happier me!

I have been overweight for most of my adult life. I tried so many different things to lose the weight with no avail. I just looked at myself in the mirror one day and said, "This is it. You will always look like this, so get used to it!"

Never in my wildest dreams did I ever think I would be this size again. I have lost 75 pounds, 7 inches in my bust and in my hips, and 11½ inches in my waist! Not to mention how good I feel. I just know I am healthier (body, mind, and soul).

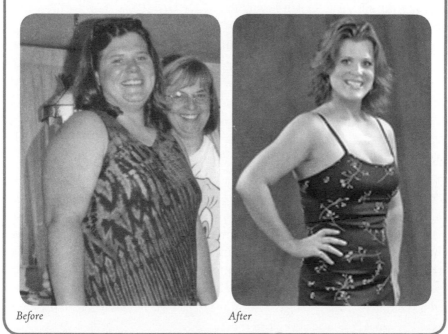

Before   *After*

All of the seasons embody an approach to wellness that you can sustain for the rest of your life. (You will note that regardless of which season these modalities are introduced, many of these wellness techniques are repeated in succeeding seasons as you build on a life-care program.)

SEASONAL FITNESS

The final piece of Fat Flush for Life is exercise. Exercise is great for many things—your heart, your lungs, your bones, and your brain. What most people don't realize is that exercise detoxifies the body, too. And that's precisely why I'm including a fitness program that specifically targets the lymphatic system to provide an "inside-out" workout. The blood has a heart to keep it pumping through your veins and arteries, but the lymphatics have only you. It is your own bodily movement—bouncing, walking, running, and stretching with your legs and arms lifting, pumping, and swinging—that keeps lymph on the move. Deep breathing and massage will also keep the lymph flowing. These forms of "detox fitness" easily and effectively push fat, waste, and toxins out of your body. You will be rewarded with enhanced weight loss, improved immunity, and smoother, sleeker skin.

The Fat Flush for Life program combines yoga, stretching, cardio, and core exercises that correspond to the seasonal diet program. In addition to increasing energy, flexibility, and strength, you'll discover how to:

- Burn surplus fat and flatten your belly
- Erase the unsightly appearance of cellulite
- Lose inches in your waist, thighs, and hips
- Rev up your metabolism by building lean muscle mass
- Enhance core stability by working the muscles deep in your abdomen, trunk, pelvis, and back
- Strengthen the immune system by targeting the lymph

Before you begin your first seasonal fitness plan, as you would with any new exercise regimen, check with your doctor first. This is important especially if you have any disabilities, ailments, or conditions such as high blood pressure, a heart condition, pregnancy, asthma, or diabetes, which might be affected by vigorous activity. If at any time while exercising, you feel any chest pain or tightness in the chest, rapid heartbeat, shortness of breath, or dizziness, stop right away. If these symptoms don't dissipate within five minutes, seek medical help. If you feel any of the exercises are beyond your current fitness level, simply use the "modify" version to better match your capability. Take it one step at a time and before you know it, you will be stepping into a whole new you.

4 SIGNATURE FAT FLUSH DIET FEATURES

No self-respecting swashbuckling buccaneer would set out in search of buried treasure without a map. Why should you?

—Sarah Ban Breathnach

FAT FLUSH IS KNOWN AS A SUPERDETOX for good reason. It details a strategy that you haven't seen in other weight loss diets—an emphasis on the most cleansing superfoods, beverages, herbs, spices, supplements, and an avoidance of high-copper and zinc-depleting foods. This unique diet formula builds vitality and strength while supporting liver, lymph, GI tract, and thyroid functions as you burn and flush out fat. Here is a showcase of the Fat Flushing staples and strategies that you will be enjoying year round.

FAT FLUSHING STAPLES
Cranberry H$_2$O
The signature Fat Flushing beverage is cranberry juice diluted with water. Cranberries are one of the highest sources of the proanthocyanidins and phenols (antioxidants) on the planet. These brightly colored phytonutrients strengthen connective tissue, protect blood vessel walls from damage by free radicals, and, based upon thousands of Fat Flushing testimonials, are responsible for cellulite- and varicose vein–free legs. Cranberry juice, a known cleanser of the urinary tract, also contains several organic acids that are potent digestion regulators.

In my experience with Fat Flushers over the past twenty years, these acids also act as fat-flushing enzymes, emulsifying and moving out stagnant lymphatic waste and fluids. They also keep the colon healthy by providing an acidic environment that is inhospitable to pathogens and allows probiotics to live happily ever after. Cranberry H$_2$O is introduced in Winter Fat Flush and should be used throughout the entire program.

Green Life Cocktail
"Going green" takes on new meaning in *Fat Flush for Life*—adding plant power to your diet in a daily Green Life Cocktail year round. Now you can drink your greens because so many folks are simply not eating them these days. Greens—leafy and dark—are nutrient packed with essential amino acids, fiber, antioxidants,

potassium, flavonoids, carotenoids, lutein and folic acid, and chlorophyll (the "green" in greens). Chlorophyll delivers more than color. It helps oxygenate the blood while providing magnesium, supports tissue growth, eliminates the negative effects of pollution, cleanses breath, acts as a natural deodorant, and roadblocks carcinogens.

The cocktail is a blend of the cleansing Cranberry H_2O with a "clean" green from either gluten-free wheatgrass or the Liver-Lovin' Formula (containing chlorophyll, artichoke, and the amino acid taurine, which boosts bile production). The probiotic natural sweetener Flora-Key is also included in the cocktail. It promotes elimination and aids the production of friendly flora that your body needs for enhanced immunity and weight loss.

Chia Seeds

Once a sacred food of ancient cultures, chia seeds have now emerged as a Fat Flushing staple. Chia seeds are considered the world's most fiber-rich food (soluble and insoluble) and the highest natural source of omega-3s, which have been proven to lower fattening hormones such as cortisol.

Chia seeds are extremely nutritionally dense, gluten free, and abundant in antioxidants, vitamin C, minerals, fiber, essential fatty acids, and protein. Just one ounce of chia seeds yields about 4.9 grams of omega-3s, more than 100 percent of the daily dose recommended by the American Heart Association; 10.6 grams of soluble fiber, more than one-third of the USDA recommended daily amount; 177 milligrams (mg) of calcium compared to 56 mg contained in a single stalk of broccoli; and 4.4 grams of protein versus 0.01 grams found in a one-ounce portion of kidney beans.

Unlike flaxseeds that need to be ground to get the full nutritional benefits, chia seeds are easily digested without the extra step of grinding. With a neutral flavor that works to enhance the taste of other foods, a couple of tablespoons of chia seeds daily are the latest addition to the Fat Flush protocol. Sprinkle them in frappés, casseroles, salads, veggies, and yogurt. The seeds retain their freshness for a long time when kept in a cool, dry area.

Slimming Oils

On a very practical level, fats improve the taste of food and help to make you feel full. Our body couldn't function without fats. Fats play a role in hormone production, oxygen transport, calcium absorption, fat-soluble mineral absorption (including vitamins A, D, E, and K), as well as detoxification. When you are on the Spring or Summer Fat Flush diets, you will be able to benefit from spritzes of olive oil for cooking and one to two tablespoons of fish and/or flaxseed oil.

The same is true for Autumn Fat Flush, with the exception of fish oil, which is substituted for another tablespoon of flaxseed oil. So, vegans and vegetarians who avoid fish should use the extra tablespoon of flaxseed oil. In Winter Fat Flush, you will use one tablespoon of olive, macadamia nut, sesame, or coconut oil as well as one tablespoon of fish or flaxseed oil.

Gamma linolenic acid (GLA) is recommended throughout the program to keep skin moist and taut and to mobilize the metabolically active brown fat. GLA is available in health food stores or can be obtained as part of the Fat Flush Kit in the GLA 90s (see resources, page 257) in the study-backed dosage I have been using with Fat Flushers for years.

Conjugated linoleic acid (CLA) is yet another part of the tried-and-true Fat Flushing arsenal due to its ability to increase your metabolism, decrease your abdominal fat, and build your muscle as well as enhance your immune system. It is no surprise that in landmark research published in the *Journal of Clinical Nutrition*, CLA was shown to reduce fat and preserve muscle tissue. In fact an average reduction of six pounds of body fat was found in the group that took CLA compared to the placebo group.[1]

Powerhouse Protein

Most of my Fat Flushers are totally surprised when they find animal protein on the menu. After all, Fat Flush is a detox diet. I quickly remind them that despite the juice cleanses popular these days, the right kind of protein is absolutely necessary to ensure that the liver can produce enough enzymes to break down toxins into water-soluble substances for excretion. Adequate protein is critical for both preventing and overcoming copper overload. Protein helps boost metabolism by stimulating thyroid function. It also assists the body in absorbing and retaining zinc—the nutrient that helps to prevent and balance copper. Zinc-rich lean beef, veal, lamb, skinless chicken or turkey, and many kinds of fish can be eaten to the tune of eight ounces or more per day. Soy products such as tofu and tempeh are limited to twice per week because of their high copper content, but two eggs can be enjoyed every day because of they are a high source of zinc.

Protein is a great source of steady energy for Fat Flushers due to its blood sugar stabilizing effect. Protein also helps relieve water-logged tissues.

When the body is deficient in protein, fluid leaks from the vascular spaces into the spaces between the cells and becomes trapped. This results in cellulite, water retention, bloating, and water weight gain.

Whey protein, especially in the form of a pure, undenatured, and unheated whey protein powder, helps with the production of the powerful antioxidant glutathione, nicknamed "the toxic waste neutralizer," which fights toxins, aging, and disease. For those who are vegan or allergic to whey, the Fat Flush Body Protein, introduced in Autumn Fat Flush, is a delicious combination of pea protein and brown rice, a suitable alternative. In the form of key amino acids, whey protein powder contains the richest glutathione building blocks. On Fat Flush for Life you can enjoy two servings of whey protein powder per day throughout the program.

Colorful Veggies and Fruits

Veggies and fruits are a cornerstone of Fat Flushing. They provide detoxifying enzymes, fiber, vitamins, minerals, and chlorophyll for radiant good health. They are also a rich source of phytochemicals, such as the carotenoids, beta-carotene, alpha-carotene, lycopene, and xanthophylls, which show great potential for lowering cancer risk and boosting the immune function to help protect against environmental pollutants.

A smart way to save money and reap higher nutrient benefits is to eat fruits and veggies that are in season. For example, you can enjoy strawberries and peas in the spring, berries and tomatoes in the summer, apples and burdock root in the fall, and end the year with grapefruit and carrots in the winter. Fat Flushers have discovered the Web site www.fruitsandveggiesmorematters.gov, a wonderful resource to find out what's in season and when.

Your daily dose is at least five veggies and two fruits in each seasonal diet. In the colder months you'll be eating starchier veggies and selected nongluten grains. Most people find that these "clean carbs," unlike the reactive carbs such as wheat, rye, barley, spelt, and kamut, do not create digestive difficulties, a metabolic meltdown, or binging. Since these foods are generally well tolerated, you will be pleasantly surprised that regardless of their calorie or carb content, you will not gain weight or adversely impact your blood sugar.

Sea Veggies

Sea vegetables such as hijiki, arame, nori, agar, kombu, and wakame contain some of the highest trace mineral content of any plant groups. These veggies are especially

---

Hold the Mercury

Sadly, due to the increasing levels of mercury, consuming such fish as swordfish, fresh and frozen tuna, mackerel, and tilefish, as well as some kinds of shellfish, needs to be regulated. If you really enjoy eating fish, I encourage you to visit www.gotmercury.org, which will provide you with an online calculator that can help you choose different types of fish and learn how much mercury you may be ingesting. In general, I am now recommending that you avoid freshwater and farm-raised fish altogether.

high in calcium, iron, and iodine—a mineral that supports thyroid function so that your metabolism will be at peak performance. Sea vegetables are also well known to be protective against environmental pollutants, especially radon, due to their sodium alginate content. Just in case you haven't quite developed your taste for these greens from the sea, a dash of Seaweed Gomasio (a seasoning with the sea veggies dulse, nori, and kombu; sesame seeds; and sea salt) will do just fine. Sea veggies are built into the menu plans, twice a week. You also have the option of using a daily dash of Seaweed Gomasio if you are not a full-fledged sea veggie lover.

Fat Flushing Supplements

I created the Fat Flush Kit to accompany the Fat Flush program. Besides a Dieters' Multi and the metabolic activator GLA-90 (which supplies 90 mg of black currant seed oil), the kit also contains my Weight Loss Formula. This formula includes key B vitamins as well as 400 mcg of chromium to help quell carb cravings. It also contains L-carnitine, methionine, inositol, and lipase to assist in digestion and metabolism of both carbs and fats. Finally the formula provides special support for the liver with its proprietary herbal blend of turmeric, dandelion root, milk thistle, Oregon grape root, and the fat-busting enzyme lipase (see resources, page 257).

FAT FLUSHING STRATEGIES
Organic Foods

The largest study of organic foods suggests that there are 40 percent more healing compounds in various organic fruits and vegetables compared to their conventional counterparts.[2] But let's face it, organic food is expensive. There are creative ways to go semiorganic while still reaping the benefits of less pesticides and chemicals. The Environmental Working Group has put together a list of the 12 Least and 12 Most Contaminated Foods. When you follow this list, you will save money, reduce your toxic load, and buy only organic when it will make a difference.

> # From the Fat Flush Grapevine
>
> Yet another little known secret is that produce is labeled with a coded sticker that tells you not only if it is organic versus conventionally grown, but if it is genetically modified (GM). The trick is to look at the number on the tiny labels. A four-digit code tells you the produce is conventionally grown. A five-digit code that begins with a 9 tells you it is organic. And last but certainly not least, a five-digit code that starts with an 8 tells you it is, in fact, genetically modified. So in this case, 8 is not great.

12 LEAST CONTAMINATED FOODS No Need to Buy Organic	12 MOST CONTAMINATED FOODS Consider Buying These Organic
1. Onions	1. Peaches
2. Avocados	2. Apples
3. Sweet corn	3. Sweet bell peppers
4. Pineapples	4. Celery
5. Mangoes	5. Nectarines
6. Asparagus	6. Strawberries
7. Sweet peas	7. Cherries
8. Kiwi	8. Pears
9. Bananas	9. Grapes, imported
10. Cabbage	10. Spinach
11. Broccoli	11. Lettuce
12. Papaya	12. Potatoes

Parcells' Clorox Bath

The Fat Flush way to help remove pesticides, bacteria, parasites, and other contaminants from food is through the Parcells' Clorox Bath. Dr. Hazel Parcells, head of the Nutrition Department at Sierra States University, discovered this food bath in the 1960s. She decided to test a theory of using Clorox as an effective food cleanser with a box of shriveled lemons that were about to be thrown out. She dropped the lemons into water mixed with some Clorox. To her delight, within thirty minutes the lemons plumped up as if they were just picked from the tree. The entire room became filled with the fragrance of fresh lemons. Dr. Parcells deduced that it was the oxygenating value of Clorox that made the difference. As the years went on, she experimented with many other types of bleach on the market, but found that the Clorox brand was the one to use for food-cleansing purposes. This formula is registered with the Smithsonian Institution.

The bath also improves the taste of foods and extends storage life by at least two weeks. Fruits and veggies taste farm fresh; leafy vegetables retain their color and crispness; meats are tenderized; and allergic responses are eliminated.

Meet a Fat Flusher for Life

Cathy G., Lake Placid, New York
48 years old; mother of two; 5-year Fat Flusher; lost 43 pounds

I had been working in the health food business for ten years, and while I had knowledge of herbs and vitamins, and tried many different diets over the years, nothing clicked as well and made more sense than Fat Flush.

I tried many different diets, but even if I lost the weight, It would come back, and it still never got rid of many of my symptoms. …and eventually gained a lot of weight again, shooting up to 170 or so, which is a lot for my small-framed 5 foot 3 inch body! I started Fat Flush in earnest right before the holidays. What an amazing journey! I've never experienced anything like it, and I lost a total of 43 pounds and 38 inches in a matter of about four to five months!

The Forum is the tool that really kept me going… There are so many wonderful people who helped me through some tough times and answered questions. I am happy to say that I look and feel better than I did at twenty-five, and fit into a solid size 4, which I never thought I could do.

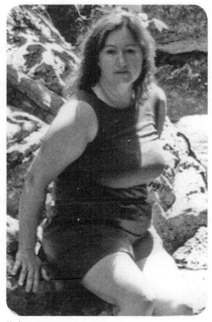

Before

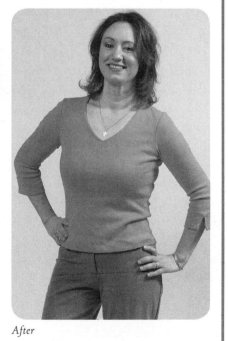

After

Dr. Parcells' recommended formula is to add exactly 1 teaspoon of Clorox bleach to 1 gallon of water, then bathe the food according to the following guidelines:

Thin-skinned fruits (such as apricots, berries, plums, peaches)	15 minutes
Leafy vegetables	15 minutes
Poultry, fish, meat, eggs	20 minutes
Thick-skinned fruits, such as apples, bananas, citrus	30 minutes
Thin-skinned root or fibrous vegetables	30 minutes

Remove the food from the bath after the allotted time is up and place it in clear water for ten minutes, then remove, rinse, and dry thoroughly. The bath can also be used as a thawing method for frozen meat (not ground meat). Soak the meat for about twenty minutes for up to five pounds, then rinse in clear water and dry as for other foods.

YOU KNOW YOU ARE A FAT FLUSHER WHEN… *you're in Whole Foods and realize that the cranberry juice is on sale, so you buy ten bottles.*

PARTING WORDS

Together, the Fat Flush food plans, fitness, and wellness practices complete a larger vision of self-care in *Fat Flush for Life*. To become a highly efficient Fat Flusher, you must embrace the fact that your body needs proper movement and wellness routines just as much as it needs healthy and detoxifying foods. There really are no hidden secrets to this. I'm going to spell out everything in detail, as these next chapters will reveal. All you need is willingness to change and a can-do attitude.

Part 2
The Pre–Fat Flush Week

5 THE PRE–FAT FLUSH DIET

THE PRE–FAT FLUSH DIET IS A 7-DAY PROGRAM designed to prepare you for what's to come and make the transition to every seasonal Fat Flush as easy as possible. I've included a smorgasbord of the best from each season—Summer Fat Flush's detoxifying fruits and veggies; Spring Fat Flush's fiber-filled, complex carbs; and Autumn and Winter's root vegetables and calcium-rich dairy. With a few twists on some old favorites, some speedy and easy recipes, and the promise of vivid flavors at every meal, you can slowly and deliciously ease through this first step of the transition into the full-fledged program.

The Pre–Fat Flush diet week is also about getting more conscious of food choices. Making the cut to eliminate some of the worst liver stressors or metabolism downers—sugar and all of its kissin' cousins such as high-fructose corn syrup and artificial sweeteners, caffeine, and trans fats—is the goal. So eliminate or cut back on foods that make you pooch and puff out, such as gum, diet soda, carbonated beverages, alcohol, beans, excessive raw foods, excess salt, processed and refined foods, and too many carbs in general. You will also be cutting back on foods and beverages that stimulate fat-promoting cortisol and insulin—such as coffee and regular teas—which can inhibit optimal weight-loss results.

A few simple changes is all it takes. Omitting all sugar and sugar substitutes (especially bloat-producing sugar alcohols such as sorbitol, maltitol, mannitol, and xylitol) will flatten your belly from the get-go. You will be motivated by instant, measurable results that will capture your attention and keep you going for the remainder of the program. Just think—you can enjoy mouthwatering dishes such as Raspberry Yogurt Crunch and Quick 'n' E-Z Spicy Shrimp—and no more bloat.

Many Fat Flushers have found that simply sticking with just one week of the Pre–Fat Flush Diet is all they need to shed a few pounds (of course, these are usually the people who only have a few pounds to lose anyway). By implementing small changes every day, such as giving up sugarless gum and diet soda, you will lose the weight and feel better all over—no more headaches, no blood sugar peaks and valleys, no foggy thinking, and of course, a no-bloat belly. You will be surprised how much incremental dietary changes will do for you in lifting your Fat Flushing confidence.

This week we are going to start slow—so relax.

Right now you can get started by loading up on powerful proteins (lean beef, fish and poultry), quality oils (flaxseed oil and olive oil), and colorful fruits and veggies while eliminating metabolism downers. Drink plenty of purifying water, and by all means don't forget to give yourself an oil change so you can fight fat with the right fat. This is the time to clear out as many unhealthy items as possible, especially packaged foods with long lists of chemical-sounding ingredients. Single-ingredient foods such as your olive oil, berries, and lean meat are keepers. The other surprising "keepers" are the spices in your pantry, because they are fat-burning flavor enhancers. Seasoning your foods with a pinch of cumin or cayenne can really boost your

> ## Turbo-charge Your Weight Loss
>
> **Say YES** to drinking more water.
> **Say YES** to using healthy oils.
> **Say YES** to vegetables.
> **Say YES** to lean protein.
> **Say YES** to fruits.
>
> ---
>
> **SAY NO** to sugar-free gum and diet sodas that can pooch out your tummy.
> **SAY NO** to sugary stuff and yeasty foods to avoid bloating.
> **SAY NO** to booze because alcohol can make you retain fluid.
> **SAY NO** to salty processed foods, since they cause fluid retention.

weight loss. These potent flavor enhancers help you steer clear of bloat-promoting preservatives, salt, and artificial additives. By the end of the week, you will be on your way to a slimmer, more relaxed, and younger-looking you.

DETERMINING YOUR GOALS

This is a good time to take a moment to determine your goals. To make lasting lifestyle adjustments, you must first identify the specific results *you* want to obtain. Weight loss? Detox? A combination of both? It is very important for you to settle on a realistic, attainable weight so that you set yourself up for resounding success. As soon as you have decided upon a measurable goal, further empower yourself by imagining that you already have achieved your future now, in the present. For weight-loss purposes, use this chart as a guide to determine your ideal weight.

> *Do not look any further! You have arrived! This is not only the best way to find the "healthy [person]" inside of you. ...It's a way of life that will make you feel and look different in ways you never dreamed possible. It's a process and it works.*
>
> —Jennifer (Fat Flush Online Fan)

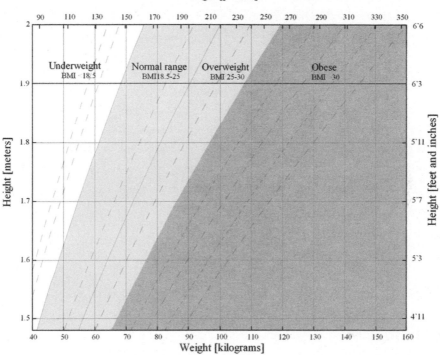

FAT FLUSH FLASH FORWARD

Now is a good time to stock up on important Fat Flush items, including those you may want to order, so that you'll be ready for the next step in your diet. For your convenience, I am recommending products that I have been using with Fat Flushers for the past fifteen years. I had to personally develop these because of my concerns about the inferior quality of raw materials and changing formulations in the marketplace. You are welcome to check out the formulas and compare them with your local health food store offerings. For your convenience, these items are available online from Uni Key Health Systems, Inc. (www.unikeyhealth.com), my official distribution center (see resources, page 257).

     Probiotic sweetener—Flora-Key
     Protein powder—Fat Flush Whey Protein Powder
     Chia seeds—Bella Chia Corp.
     Flaxseed and/or fish oil
     Liver-Lovin' Formula
     Fat Flush Kit
     CLA

A Gentle Reminder—Especially for the Pre–Fat Flush Diet

In the Pre–Fat Flush Diet's 7-Day Meal Planner, you will find a sample week that includes the right proteins, fats, and carbs as well as Fat Flushing herbs and spices.

- Menu plans are completely optional. If following a structured plan is not for you, feel free to create your own fabulous Fat Flush–friendly meals and snacks that follow the Pre–Fat Flush diet guidelines.
- Recipes noted with an asterisk (*) appear in chapter 21.
- Lunches, dinners, and snacks are interchangeable within the same day.
- Don't forget to drink at least eight ounces of water between each meal and each snack daily.

PRE–FAT FLUSH 7-DAY MEAL PLANNER

DAY 1

Breakfast
   1 cup berries
   2 poached eggs
   1 slice multigrain toast
   1 cup coffee or herbal tea

Snack
   1 glass V8 juice
   4 walnut halves

Lunch
   Tuna salad on mixed greens with 1 table-
      spoon of mayo plus sprouts, red
      onions, and celery
   5 brown rice crackers

Snack
   1 ounce string cheese
   1 apple

Dinner
   Grilled beef burger with sliced onions and
      parsley
   Warm green beans
   Baked potato with 1 tablespoon of
      flaxseed oil
   1 cup herbal tea

   *Fat Flush on the Fly: Applegate Farms
   Organic Beef Burgers*

DAY 2

Breakfast
1 serving Break of Dawn Oatmeal* (page 205)
1 cup coffee or herbal tea

Snack
Red bell pepper sticks with ¼ cup of hummus

Fat Flush on the Fly: *Tribe Hummus*

Lunch
Roast Beef and Veggie Wrap with roast beef in a multigrain tortilla with veggies and Dijon mustard
Mixed green salad with apple cider vinegar and 1 tablespoon of olive oil

Fat Flush on the Fly: *Applegate Farms Roast Beef Slices*

Snack
Raspberry Yogurt Crunch made with 1 cup of plain low-fat yogurt, ½ cup of raspberries, and 1 tablespoon of toasted sunflower seeds

Dinner
Quick 'n' E-Z Spicy Shrimp* (page 217)
½ cup cooked brown rice pasta
Steamed snow peas with 1 tablespoon of sesame seeds and 1 tablespoon of flaxseed oil
1 cup herbal tea

Timesaver Tip! *Save leftover shrimp for Day 3's Lunch.*

DAY 3

Breakfast
Egg, Portobello, and Spinach Tower* (page 206)
1 slice multigrain toast
1 cup coffee or herbal tea

Snack
Pear slices with 1 tablespoon of almond butter

Lunch
Leftover Quick 'n' E-7 Spicy Shrimp*
Baby greens salad with black olives and 2 tablespoons of Herbal Dijon Vinaigrette* (page 238)

Fat Flush on the Fly: *No time to make salad dressing? Try Bragg Ginger & Sesame Salad Dressing.*

Snack
Banana Bliss
½ cup ricotta cheese with sliced bananas

Dinner
Can't Resist Chick 'n' Spinach Chili* (page 208)
½ cup steamed brown rice
Steamed Brussels sprouts with 1 tablespoon of flaxseed oil and nutmeg
1 cup herbal tea

Timesaver Tip! *Save leftover chili for Day 4's Lunch.*

DAY 4

Breakfast
2-Egg Veggie Scramble with red, yellow, and orange bell peppers
½ multigrain English muffin
1 cup coffee or herbal tea

Snack
Cucumber spears with salsa

Lunch
Leftover Can't Resist Chick 'n Spinach Chili*
½ cup brown rice
Cherry tomato, chopped parsley, and cilantro salad with freshly squeezed lime juice and 1 tablespoon of olive oil

Snack
1 cup plain low-fat yogurt with 1 chopped apple and ground cinnamon

Dinner
Grilled sirloin rubbed with garlic and cayenne
Green and yellow squash medley with rosemary
Garden salad with lemon and 1 tablespoon of flaxseed oil
1 cup herbal tea

DAY 5

Breakfast
1 slice multigrain toast with 2 tablespoons of peanut butter
1 cup coffee or herbal tea

Snack
1 nectarine
4 walnut halves

Lunch
Dragon Bowl Salad* (page 219) with canned salmon and 2 tablespoons of Herbal Dijon Vinaigrette* (page 238)
5 brown rice crackers

Snack
2 plums
1 ounce Swiss cheese

Dinner
Grilled lamb chops with ground cumin and cinnamon
½ cup steamed garden peas
Eggplant sautéed in 1 tablespoon of olive oil with garlic
1 cup herbal tea

DAY 6

Breakfast
1 cup cottage cheese with berries
½ multigrain English muffin
1 cup coffee or herbal tea

Snack
2 hard-boiled eggs smashed with 1
   tablespoon of mayo plus celery and
   cayenne

Lunch
2 turkey hot dogs with Dijon mustard
Baby spinach salad with lemon and 1
   tablespoon of olive oil
7 blue corn tortilla chips

Fat Flush on the Fly: Applegate Farms
   Organic Uncured Turkey Hot Dogs

Snack
1 peach
7 almonds

Dinner
Grilled herbed chicken breast with lime
   juice and cilantro
Steamed baby carrots with dill
1 cup herbal tea

Timesaver Tip! Grill an extra chicken breast
   for Day 7's Lunch.

Fat Flush on the Fly: Plain supermarket rotisseried chicken

DAY 7

Breakfast
1 whole-grain waffle with 2 tablespoons of
   peanut butter
1 cup coffee or herbal tea

Fat Flush on the Fly: Van's Wheat Free
   Homestyle Waffles

Snack
½ cup unsweetened applesauce with
   ground cinnamon
4 walnut halves

Lunch
Dragon Bowl Salad* (page 219) topped
   with leftover chicken and 2 tablespoons of Herbal Dijon Vinaigrette*
   (page 238)
Handful of blue corn chips

Snack
1 cup plain low-fat yogurt with 6 strawberries and 1 tablespoon of toasted
   sunflower seeds

Dinner
Grilled turkey burger with fennel
1 small sweet potato
Steamed broccoli with 1 tablespoon of
   flaxseed oil
1 cup herbal tea

Fat Flush on the Fly: Applegate Farms
   Organic Turkey Slices

6 PRE–FAT FLUSH WELLNESS PROGRAM

A CRUCIAL COMPONENT of your Fat Flushing journey is acknowledging the mind-body connection. Repressed emotions and self-sabotaging patterns can become embedded in the cells, triggering behavior that can impede your weight-loss progress.

I firmly believe that seven out of ten women fail their diets due to a lack of support. Support empowers individuals to cope with the emotional, social, and spiritual issues associated with foods. I have seen this time and time again on my online Forum (www.annlouiseforum.com), where one of my community members wrote, "I would have never in my wildest imagination conceived that I could be so fed, so fortified, so supported, so connected to an online community."

NURTURING SUPPORT

Women, in particular, benefit from the support of others in achieving not only their weight-loss goals but in being able to handle all aspects of life. A landmark study from UCLA proves something that my Forum members have already suspected: a unique friendship forms between women. Your circle of friends always makes life brighter, funnier, and the tough times easier.

The researchers at UCLA have demonstrated that women who are under stress produce brain chemicals that open them up to making and maintaining friendships with other women. One of the study's leading researchers, Laura Cousin Klein, PhD, explains that before this study, it was generally assumed that when a person experiences stress, the hormones released created a fight-or-flight response. But women have a distinct response to stress. "In fact," says Dr. Klein, "it seems that when the hormone oxycotin is released as part of the stress responses in a woman, it buffers the fight-or-flight response and encourages her to tend children and gather with other women instead." Men do not have this response because of the high amounts of testosterone they produce when they are under stress. So when men are stressed they tend to go off by themselves, and when women are stressed they gather other women around them.[1]

Friends may be helping us live longer and better. And, when it comes to weight loss, there's no reason to do it alone, anymore. My online Forum community is one of the most nurturing, supportive, and encouraging places to call home. I invite you to visit the Forum and see for yourself just how wonderfully supportive and encouraging these Fat Flushers can be.

After six months on Fat Flush, I was addicted to the 24/7 online messaging board called "The Forum." All of the people on it are great and very helpful and supportive. We feel like best friends and talk to each other and joke with each other every day.

—Nina, Fat Flush Fan

FLOWER POWER

I have found that as you detox your physical body, buried emotions start to come up (impatience, exhaustion, discouragement, frustration, anxiety, boredom). I will be suggesting a flower remedy for each season to counter these emotions.

Flower remedies are a kind of vibrational or energy medicine, similar to homeopathic remedies that offset the emotional turbulence that can be the root of physical disorders. The Bach Flower Remedies represent a form of psychotherapy in a bottle. Developed in the 1930s by Edward Bach, an English physician, the most renowned formula, "Rescue Remedy," is a five-flower combo that is used to help alleviate trauma, whether emotional, physical, or psychological.

MASSAGE

You can count on massage as an advanced detox technique to be used year round. Most people mistakenly regard massage as a luxury. It's not. Studies show that a massage can stimulate nearly 80 percent of stagnant lymph back into circulation. When you target the areas that have the highest concentration of lymph vessels, you can boost lymph flow by twentyfold, dramatically enhancing the elimination of fats and toxins. The lymph-rich areas to stimulate are: the arms, neck, face, and chest.

It is not uncommon, particularly during the extreme detox portion of Summer Fat Flush, to experience a "cleansing crisis" in the form of short-lived headaches, fatigue, muscle aches, and pains. A massage can alleviate these symptoms while supporting your overall health. In the autumn, winter, and spring, when your fitness program includes strength-training, muscle building, increased aerobic and core exercises, a massage can help relieve sore muscles as well as reduce pain by releasing endorphins. Throughout the entire program you can take advantage of one of the primary and long-term benefits of massage—stress relief. I've talked before about how stress plays a major role in weight gain. Massage helps drive down belly-fattening levels of cortisol, lowering stress and aiding you on the way to a slimmer and happier you.

Go ahead. Relax with a massage without feeling guilty. There is also nothing more energizing and liberating than clearing negative emotions, assessing the current physical state of your body to address major underlying causes, and cleansing out toxins, while pampering yourself in the process. You will be rewarded with a brighter spirit and healthier body, so open up to welcome the wonderful changes right around the corner.

WARMING UP FOR FAT FLUSH WELLNESS

Before you begin the actual wellness protocols, prepare yourself emotionally for your new beginning. Infusing your system with the Bach Flower Remedy Walnut will be very supportive as you begin to clean out your refrigerator, leave your old habits behind, and prepare yourself for your Fat Flushing adventure. Walnut is especially designed to help with adjusting to transitional periods of life. It helps to resist powerful, outside influences and overcome the instability that can occur in the important first phase of a new beginning. This will help to offset negative influences and allow for a more tranquil and peaceful mind-set that will ease your journey.

I suggest that you take four drops of Walnut in eight ounces of water four times per day and sip it at intervals throughout the day. It can also be absorbed on the skin (such as on your wrists or other pulse points) and even in your bathwater.

> *The Fat Flush Wellness Plan helped continue my Fat Flush–fueled success by introducing me to aromatherapy baths—how can you not love a plan that says you gotta take a nice long soaking bath three times a week? In addition, lymph massages and the workouts have helped me keep my skin tight and toned. No saggy-baggy skin for me, thank you very much!*
>
> —Charli, Fat Flush Fan

Heal to Reveal

Now you are ready to perform a healing ceremony—your own personal cleansing ritual. This will help you to break the bonds of the past just as the Walnut will open you to a new direction and reveal a new image of yourself. Let's get started.

Get some paper and find a photo of yourself at your heaviest. You know, that shot of yourself that you would *never* let anyone see.

Step 1: List your habits that you feel have sabotaged your efforts to maintain your ideal body image. Things like late-night snacks, trips through the fast-food lane, eating a carton of ice cream when you are feeling blue (or just because it's there), making 101 excuses not to exercise—you get the idea. Use as many pieces of paper as it takes (no one but you will ever see this list).

Step 2: Take out some more paper and give yourself permission to get angry and/or sad. Start to write down your negative feelings—everything from being upset that your husband leaves the toilet seat up every single time to that kid in third grade who teased you. Sometimes you may feel the urge to write a note directed to another person—do it. Use as much time and paper as it takes to air out all the things that cause you to feel negative. Even if you don't know why you are feeling a certain way—say, overwhelmed—then just write down the word. Get all of that hurt, all of the anger, all of those negative feelings out on paper.

Step 3: Next, get that photo.

Step 4: Now burn it all! If you have a fireplace, toss it in; if not, tear up the papers and burn them piece by piece in an ashtray or in a metal can outside. Whatever is the safest way to reduce these things to ash (without burning the house down)—do it.

Step 5: Okay, now breathe. Close your eyes and breathe in through your nose and then slowly out through your mouth. That old you is gone. Keep your eyes closed and visualize the you that you long to be.

Keeping in Touch with Yourself

Now that you have a clear image of your future self, I want to tell you about a power tool that you will be using during your journey—journaling.

A cornerstone of the Fat Flush process is daily journaling, and now is the perfect time to begin recording what you eat, how you feel, and what measurable results you obtain. Fat Flushers find that journaling is also a great stress reliever where they can let off steam from the daily grind. Find a quiet place with relaxing music and/or scented candles to record and release your stressors on the written page. Consider this your sacred sounding board.

Whether you pick up *The Fat Flush Journal and Shopping Guide*, take an old notebook, or simply go online, journaling is a lifelong habit that will keep you on track.

PRE–FAT FLUSH FITNESS PLAN

JUST AS THE PRE–FAT FLUSH DIET IS DESIGNED to transition you into full-fledged Fat Flushing, the Pre–Fat Flush Fitness Plan will help you ease into the Fat Flushing fitness regimens, regardless of which season you begin. If you are new to fitness or haven't exercised in a while, it's imperative that this is where you start. If you're already a devoted exerciser, you should still read through this chapter. It offers valuable tips on the proper way to warm up and cool down for cardio workouts, how to monitor the intensity of your workouts, and how to begin rebounding, which is a cornerstone of Fat Flush fitness and just about the best cardio workout you'll ever get.

Rebounding is a form of cardio exercise that stimulates the lymph. The vertical motion of rebounding on a mini-trampoline or "rebounder" is the single best way to cleanse the lymphatic system because the up-and-down jumping motion parallels the way lymph nodes also operate, opening and closing vertically. Your cells get a deep squeeze from all that bouncing, which helps move toxins out. No other exercise that I know of yields the dimple-dashing, cellulite-slashing benefits regular rebounding offers. It is virtually an "excuse-proof exercise" because it can be done anywhere, year round. Other exercises that promote the efficient and smooth flow of lymph throughout the body are Yoga-Quickies and walking, which are all discussed in this chapter and will be continued through all of the seasons.

I recommend that you follow the Pre–Fat Flush Fitness Plan for two to four weeks before jumping into the fitness plan for the season you are in.

Pre–Fat Flush Workout Summary
> **Yoga-Quickies** (*5 to 10 minutes, 5 days a week*)
> Yoga-Quickie Belly Breathing
> Yoga-Quickie Calming Breath
> Yoga-Quickie Poses (1 to 5)

Pre–Fat Flush Cardio Workout (*15 to 25 minutes, 5 days a week*)
> Workout 1—Basic Walkout for Treadmill
> Workout 2—Ultralight Rebounding Routine

YOU KNOW YOU ARE A FAT FLUSHER WHEN... you have a rebounder (mini-trampoline) sitting in front of your TV.

YOGA-QUICKIES

Duration: 5 to 10 minutes
>*Frequency:* 5 days a week
>*Targets:* Lymphatic system, thyroid, muscle tightness and tension
>*Body-Shaping Tools:* Yoga mat optional

This is a short, five- to ten-minute yoga session interspersed with postures and breathing exercises known to stimulate the lymphatics and thyroid, activate blood flow, and aid in digestion. The thyroid gland, which is adjacent to the windpipe, can be stimulated significantly just by doing some basic breathing exercises. In addition, many of the poses will give your body an internal massage and help to flush the lymphatic fluid throughout the entire body.

A Yoga-Quickie can be done anywhere or anytime. Just select at least two of the exercises (and more if you have time) and before you know it you'll be more limber, calmer, and able to handle stress better than ever.

Yoga-Quickie Belly Breathing

This simple breathing technique starts by contracting the diaphragm; this places pressure on the abdominals, which causes the lungs to expand, thereby encouraging lymphatic flow. When you practice Belly Breathing, you are helping to detoxify the lymph and boost cellular metabolism by elevating oxygen in your cells. This makes Belly Breathing a surprisingly powerful weight-loss aid, plus it clears your head—no more foggy thinking. The very movement of contracting and expanding your abdomen works to tighten and flatten your belly.

Begin by placing one hand on your belly and another on your chest. Take a deep breath in through your nose, and on the inhale, feel your belly rise higher than your chest. Now exhale slowly through your mouth while contracting your abdominals and completely releasing all of the air in your lungs. Elongate your breath as you exhale. The exhale breath should last twice as long as the inhale.

Calming Breath

This type of breathing is often called "Whisper Breath" and is excellent for those of us who need to de-stress a bit. By breathing slowly and deeply, you are able to release tension throughout your body and lower your heart rate.

Breathe in through your nose and then out through your throat, making a sort of "ahhh" sound against the back of your throat on the exhale. Keep your breath even and regulated as in Belly Breathing.

YOGA-QUICKIE POSES

Although the Yoga-Quickie Poses are great for stimulating the lymphatics as well as the thyroid gland, you will need to check with your doctor before starting if you have neck and/or shoulder injuries. Some of the basic yoga poses shown are contraindicated for these conditions. Remember if something doesn't feel right, just don't do it.

1. Lymph Bridge

Duration: 15 seconds while practicing Belly Breathing; do 5 times

This posture is a backbend and a gentle inversion. It is designed to move the hard-to-reach lymphatics that are adjacent to the intestinal tract.

Lie on your back with your knees bent and your feet directly underneath your knees. Make sure your feet are placed about hip width apart. Lay your arms directly at your sides, palms facing down. Lift your hips into the air so that your weight is on your shoulders and feet. Without straining your neck and back, try to raise your belly button as high as you can and tighten your core. Your hips should form a straight line all the way to your shoulders. Lift your hips as high as you can without placing undue pressure on your neck and lower back.

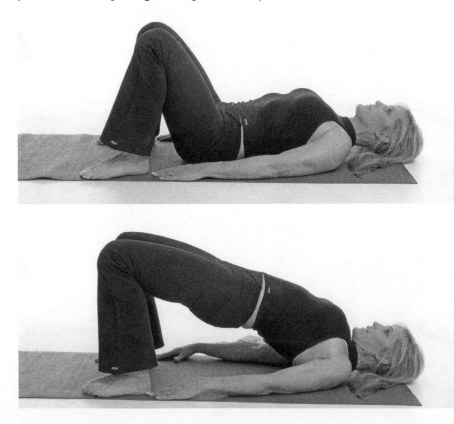

Modification: If you have weak core muscles, this pose will be somewhat challenging to hold at first. To adapt the pose to your comfort level, you can easily slide a blanket or a yoga block underneath your hips and/or shoulders for added support wherever you feel it's needed.

2. Boat Pose

Duration: 5 to 10 seconds while doing Belly Breathing; do 3 times

This pose helps to gently nudge toxins out of the kidneys. It is also good for strengthening and firming up the abdominal region.

Sit on the floor with your hands on the floor behind your hips. Straighten your spine through the top of the torso. Lean back slightly without rounding your back. Engage the core and lift your feet off the floor while slowly trying to straighten your legs.

Modify: Again, if your core muscles are weak, instead of lifting and straightening your legs, bend your knees and grasp your legs.

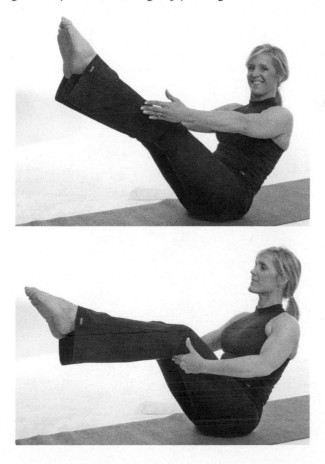

3. Cobra

Duration: 15 seconds while practicing Calming Breath; do 2 times

This pose helps to elongate and stretch muscles that affect stomach positioning, thereby helping to improve digestion, which can reduce bloat.

Lie on your abdomen with your legs together. Place your hands, palms down, right beside your chest, keeping your elbows close to the body. Roll your eyes upward toward the ceiling, allowing your head and chest to arch back slowly, and hold this position.

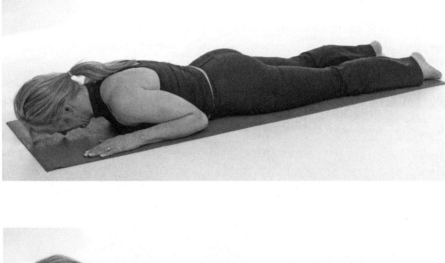

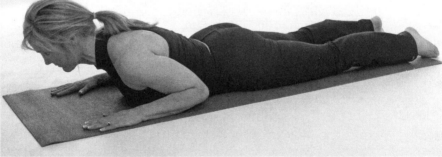

4. Downward Facing Dog

Duration: 10 seconds while practicing Belly Breathing or Calming Breath; do 2 times

This pose brings fresh blood and oxygen to your head and your stomach area, clearing out the cobwebs, relieving stiffness, and aiding digestion.

Start out on all fours, place your hands with fingers spread on the floor directly underneath your shoulders. Make sure your knees are directly under your hips. Turn your toes under, lift your hips up and straighten your legs into an upside-down V shape. To come out of the pose, bend your knees and return to all fours.

Modification: If you have tight hips and/or flexibility issues, this pose can be modified by bending your knees or placing your feet two to three feet apart.

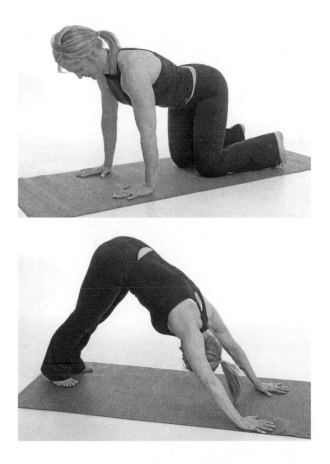

5. Corpse Pose

Duration: 3 minutes while practicing Belly Breathing or Calming Breath

This pose is the ultimate for relaxation and is proven to help lower stress-induced cortisol levels, which helps to eliminate belly fat. It's all about letting go, using either Belly Breathing or Calming Breath.

Simply lie down on the floor on your back, with your arms at your sides and your palms facing up. Relax your spine, neck, shoulders, and hips so that your feet naturally fall out to the side. Close your eyes and practice the breathing exercises.

Modification: If you feel any discomfort, place a pillow underneath your knees, neck, or lower back.

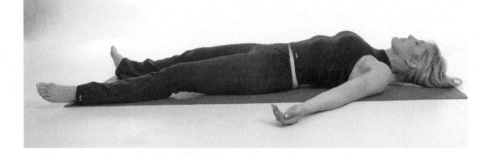

GETTING READY FOR CARDIO WORKOUT: WARM UP AND COOL DOWN

Always warm up before you stretch and exercise. Stretching and exercising when your muscles are cold puts you at greater risk for muscle pulls or muscle tears. The goal of the warm-up phase is to get the blood flowing, the heart pumping, the muscles warm. To begin, walk at a nice, easy pace for the first five to ten minutes. Then, do a few gentle stretches to prepare the body for a more vigorous workout.

The cool-down phase is just as important as the warm-up. You should never just abruptly stop after an intense workout. Your heart rate and blood pressure can go south dramatically and can make you dizzy and lightheaded. Cool down at the end of your workout by walking at a slow pace for five to ten minutes. For added flexibility, more stretching can be incorporated during this cool-down phase.

Warm-Up Stretches

Quadriceps Stretch

Duration: Hold this stretch for 15 seconds or more. Relax and repeat with other leg.

Standing with your feet together, grab either your right ankle or calf with your right hand and lift it back toward your rear. As you pull your leg up, keep your knee in line with your hips. You should feel the pull along the front of your thigh and hip.

Modification: If flexibility is limited, you can place your foot on the back of a chair or step to perform the same stretch.

Standing Hamstring Stretch

Duration: 15 seconds; do 2 times

Place one heel on a chair, with the knee slightly bent while you keep the other leg slightly bent on the floor. Bend forward at the hips with a straight back until you feel the stretch in the back of the raised leg. Try to lean further forward while fully straightening the leg on the chair. Hold for 15 seconds. Relax and repeat with other leg.

Calf Stretch

Duration: 15 seconds; do 2 times

Stand in an upright position facing a wall at an arm's length distance. Lean toward the wall, then step one foot forward with a bent knee, and extend the other leg backward one foot, straightening the back leg while pressing back into your heel. Hold this stretch for 15 seconds. Most of the weight should be placed on your back leg. Relax and repeat with the other leg.

PRE–FAT FLUSH CARDIO WORKOUT

The goal with these Pre–Fat Flush cardio workouts is simply to get you moving with some basic walking and rebounding, so have fun and take it easy.

Cardio Workout 1—Walking

Duration: 25 minutes
Frequency: 5 days a week
Targets: Cardiovascular and lymphatic systems
Body-Shaping Tools: Walking shoes

In fact, walking is one if the easiest cardiovascular exercises you can do to improve your overall fitness. Research presented at the American Heart Association showed women who walked at a brisk pace for 70 minutes a week (or

10 minutes a day) reported 18 percent more energy after six months than those who were more sedentary. They also felt that brain fogginess had lifted and their thinking had much more clarity. Another perk was enhanced self-confidence. They complained of less aches and pains and their daily tasks became much easier to complete. Walking about 20 minutes, three or four times a week, provides the same results, the study found.[1]

Walking Tips

- Walking uphill uses the muscles in the front of your thigh and in your buttocks, burning an extra 3 to 5 calories per minute over walking on a level surface. Walking hills will raise your heart rate, breathing, and exertion level, as more muscles are used.
- Use the Rate of Perceived Exertion Scale or Target Heart Rate Chart to monitor your exercise intensity (see page 57).
- Stop if you feel faint or dizzy.
- Wear well-fitting shoes that are designed for walking. Replace your walking shoes every seven to eight months or 500 miles.
- Make sure to pump your arms vigorously. This promotes the removal of toxic waste via the lymph, especially the thoracic duct along the spine.
- To keep track of your pace, try using a pedometer and increase your steps daily during your 20-minute workout. Pedometers are sold at most sporting goods stores or check online at www.walking.about.com.
- Modify your Walkout workout according to your fitness level. If you need more recovery time, take it. If the intensity intervals are too long, walk as long as you can and rest. Add a few minutes to your workout schedule each week to progress.

MONITORING WORKOUT INTENSITY

To ensure that you don't overdo it, use the Rate of Perceived Exertion Scale or Target Heart Rate Chart to monitor your aerobic exercise intensity. In Pre–Fat Flush, you want to exert on a scale of 3 to 6. As you progress into the succeeding seasons, your level of exertion will fluctuate both higher and lower based on the amount of Clean Carbs you'll be consuming.

The easiest way to monitor the intensity of your cardio workouts is to use the Rate of Perceived Exertion Scale, which requires you to listen to your body and gauge how vigorously you are working, according to how you feel.

You usually can compare the Rate of Perceived Exertion with your heart rate. When doing intervals in Winter, Spring, Summer, and Fall Fat Flush, you can

Rate of Perceived Exertion Scale

1–2	*Very, very light exertion*—I could do this in my sleep.
3	*Very moderate exertion*—This is like a walk around the park with my dog while talking on my cell phone, too.
4–5	*Moderate*—I'm starting to feel like I'm getting a workout.
6–7	*Somewhat hard*—This is getting to be work, but I'm up for it and, hopefully, I won't feel too sore tomorrow.
8	*Hard*—I am finally breaking a sweat, and my adrenaline is flowing.
9	*Very hard*—I am breathing very heavily. I don't know how much longer I can keep this up!
10	*Very, very hard*—I'm at my maximum effort and am ready for a cool-down.

use either the Rate of Perceived Exertion or the Heart Rate Chart to figure out what your aerobic training zone should be.

Targeting Your Heart Rate

To measure your heart rate, take your pulse at your wrist or neck, using your index fingers and middle fingers. (Don't use your thumb to take your heart rate because it has its own pulse.) Count the beats for 10 seconds and multiply by 6. If you take your pulse at the neck, be careful not to press too hard, as this can shut off blood flow and make you dizzy and lightheaded.

Target Heart Rate Chart

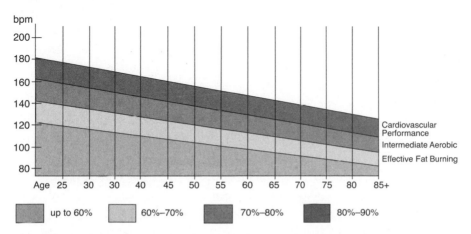

This Heart Rate Chart is based on your maximum heart rate according to your age.

People who are just starting an exercise program should start at 50 percent of their target heart rate (THR) and gradually build up as they become more fit. Moderate exercisers should stay between 50 to 70 percent of their THR. Avid exercisers and athletes can exercise between 50 to 85 percent of their THR.

GETTING STARTED WITH REBOUNDING

As simple as it seems, rebounding is one of the most efficient forms of exercise, ever. And, you don't even have to break a sweat to see and feel results. You'll have tighter abdominals, improved skin tone, and a higher muscle-to-fat ratio with less cellulite—all in the privacy of your own home. Researchers have documented improvements in balance, coordination, energy, metabolism, and even arthritis relief. NASA studies suggest rebounding is almost 70 percent more effective than jogging for calorie burning and also found rebounding as the best exercise to build bone density and possibly reverse osteoporosis.[2]

If you have never tried rebounding before, you may want to purchase a rebounder that comes with a bar attachment for added support and stability. Taking it slow at first will help you to develop balance and get your bearings, so to speak. (You may be surprised by how powerful rebounding is, which is why you will be starting with only 10 minutes. If you feel that is excessive, then cut back to 5 minutes.) Once you get acclimated to rebounding, however, you will love it. It is a very powerful workout that is also good for the cardiovascular system.

Rebounding Reminders

- Invest in a quality rebounder (see resources, page 259). Some of the less expensive models won't support more than 200 pounds of weight. A sturdy one will last you about ten years.
- If balance is a problem or you are recovering from any type of an injury, consider purchasing a rebounder with a stabilizing bar that comes as a separate attachment.
- Wear loose, comfortable clothing and cross-training shoes for better traction and ankle support.
- Remember to breathe in deeply through your nose. The more oxygen you take in and utilize, the more fat you burn.
- You can sit on the rebounder and bounce (or have someone else do the bouncing for you) and still receive benefits.
- Rebounding will stimulate lymphatic drainage, so be sure to drink all of your Cranberry H_2O and extra water (if needed) to continue the flushing process.

CARDIO WORKOUT 2—ULTRALIGHT REBOUNDING

Duration: 10 minutes
Frequency: Five days a week
Targets: Cardiovascular and lymphatic systems
Body-Shaping Tools: Rebounder

Always begin rebounding with a warm-up. A basic warm-up consists of light, gentle bouncing and/or marching for 1 minute. Bounce in the center of the rebounder for balanced weight distribution. Always cool down for 1 minute by gradually lessening the workout intensity before getting off your rebounder.

Warm-up—8 minutes
Walking slowly in place, raising your legs as high as you can
Cardio Phase—8 minutes total
    Light Bounce—3 minutes
        A gentle bounce with feet together or apart
    Jumping Jack Bounce—3 minutes
        A gentle bounce bringing feet together and apart and raising arms together
        and apart in a jumping jack motion
    Heel-Jack Bounce—2 minutes
        A bounce starting with feet together, then flex the foot and take one heel
        out, tap the rebounder and then bring the foot back. Then, repeat move
        with opposite foot.
Cool-down—1 minutes
Walking slowly in place, raising your legs as high as you can
Total Workout Time: 10 minutes, including warm-up and cool-down

THE BIG PICTURE

No matter how you exercise, no matter what program you follow, the key to exercise is regularity. As long as you make movement a part of your life, you'll help keep lymph moving, muscles toned, and joints flexible. Exercise is lifelong activity.

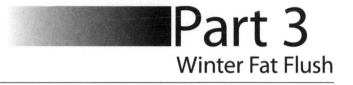

Part 3
Winter Fat Flush

8 WINTER FAT FLUSH DIET

The best and safest thing is to keep a balance in your life,
acknowledge the great powers around us and in us. If you can do
that, and live that way, you are really a wise man.

—Euripides (Greek playwright, ca. 480–406 BC)

WELCOME TO WINTER FAT FLUSH. This harmonious diet and detox approach will support you in harsher and dryer weather when you are generally less active yet still want to maintain a gentle detox momentum. You are about to embark on a journey during which you will not only lose weight; you'll achieve remarkable health benefits, such as lower cholesterol, balanced glucose levels, normal liver enzymes, thyroid improvement, better regularity, and enhanced immunity with fewer colds, viruses, and flu. You will have greater control of your food choices and be empowered with an awareness of how your body reacts to certain foods and how certain foods react to your body.

Winter is the season when your body naturally slows down, and the physical and psychological stressors of cold weather, holidays, and overwork can exhaust your kidneys and adrenals. This can cause such symptoms as:

- An inability to deal with stress
- Low stamina
- Frequent pain or weakness in the knees or lower back
- A craving for salt or addiction to sweets
- Difficulty in waking up and getting going in the morning

It's important during the cold winter months to replenish your system and conserve energy, eat warming foods, and build immunity to help regenerate and renew your kidneys and adrenals. To accomplish this, your Winter Fat Flush diet will include limited amounts of dairy and hypoallergenic or "Clean Carbs" such as starchy veggies—sweet potatoes, butternut squash, and acorn squash—and root veggies such as turnips, parsnips, beets, and potatoes. This is the time to take advantage of richer, more sustaining and nourishing foods such as high-quality meats, nuts, seeds, cheese, and warming winter grains.

One especially delicious feature of Winter Fat Flush is the wide variety of slimming oils you can use, particularly macadamia nut oil. Macadamia nut oil has developed a reputation as the world's healthiest oil due to its high level of good monounsaturated fats—in excess of 80 percent. Not even olive oil is that good! Macadamia nut oil has a smoke point about twice that of olive oil, meaning you can use it for a huge range of cooking, including frying, baking, and basting. Best of all, macadamia nut oil tastes great—an exquisite nutty flavor and aroma. Plus you can warm up with a tablespoon of either coconut oil, sesame oil, olive oil, or macadamia nut oil as part of the meal plan in addition to a tablespoon of either flaxseed or fish oil for your daily omega-3 fix.

As in the Pre–Fat Flush Diet, you can again include carefully selected, healthy convenience foods noted on the menu called Fat Flush on the Fly (see page XX). They allow for convenience in the program but also add a healthy dose of sodium. And while we are on the subject of salt, let me tell you there is as much misunderstanding about sodium as there was once about fats. Sodium is essential to good digestion, the acid/alkaline balance, and the lymph and blood fluid. Without enough sodium in the system, calcium can be deposited in the joints, creating joint problems such as arthritis. Organic sodium is a potent neutralizer of excessive acidity. The USDA Food Guidelines suggest 2,400 mg per day is a safe sodium intake for most adults. This is why you will occasionally find turkey bacon (a "Legal Cheat" that contains 200 mg of sodium per slice) in the meal plans.

Many women, particularly those with high blood pressure or who retain fluid and bloat easily, need to watch salt intake more carefully. If you are one of these women, consider keeping your sodium intake to about 1,000 mg. On the other hand, if you suffer from low blood pressure, then by all means make sure that you consume about one teaspoon of salt per day. In fact, in a study published in the *Journal of General Internal Medicine*, researchers found that salt is actually important to maintaining a healthy heart.[1]

Teas and Herbs that Cleanse, Heal, and Relax

Nettle tea is the wintertime herbal tea of choice. If any of the symptoms that relate to the kidneys and adrenals resonate with you, I suggest you use nettle tea to complement any of the other Fat Flushing beverages in Winter Fat Flush. Nettle tea is rich in alkalizing minerals that are good for kidney cleansing.

Specific kidney- and adrenal-protecting herbs include deglycyrrhizinated licorice root, which acts as a tonic for the adrenal glands and helps regulate cortisol, and rehmannia, a well-respected kidney strengthener that encourages normal fluid elimination, facilitates a healthy response to stress, and fortifies the system against harsh winter assaults.

Suddenly, and for the first time in years, I feel in control of what goes into my body and not controlled by the foods or beverages in front of me. Isn't life all about choices anyway? So glad I chose Fat Flush. Here's to… a new lifestyle of balance and health.

—*Jennifer, Fat Flush Online Fan*

WINTER FAT FLUSHING SUPERSTAR FOODS

So long, hunger. As you step into Winter Fat Flush, you will be nourished by Fat Flushing Superfoods that will banish bloat, rev up metabolism, and speed up fat loss. I've even added some alcohol—in moderation of course—to lift your spirits during these long winter months. (It would be a great idea to put a copy of the protocol on your PDA or your cell phone, or just make a make a copy and tape it to your fridge and/or carry it with you when shopping). At a glance you will find the benefits, brands, and bodily consumption recommendations for each staple and food category as it is introduced. Each succeeding season has its own Superstar Foods list, and while many of the staples will remain constant through all four seasons, you will find that each list is unique based on your bodily needs for that period of time. **Each of the food equivalents is interchangeable with all others listed in the same group.** In the portions given, these provide the same vitamins, minerals, enzymes, antioxidants, fatty acids, and amino acids—the very things your body needs for purification and accelerated weight loss.

> **YOU KNOW YOU ARE A FAT FLUSHER WHEN…** you have commandeered the entire bottom shelf of your refrigerator for your eggs, fresh veggies, and leftovers.

Cranberry H_2O

Benefits: The cranberry component helps balance pH to suppress hunger; it also conquers cellulite, fights water retention, and draws fatty wastes from the lymphatic system. Rich source of antioxidants for cardio, liver, and urinary tract health.

Brands: Unsweetened cranberry juice (no sugar, artificial sweeteners, other juices, or corn syrup added)—Knudsen's, Trader Joe's, Mountain Sun, Tree of Life, Whole Foods, Lakewood, or unsweetened cranberry juice concentrate—Knudsen's, Tree of Life

For those allergic to cranberry juice, see alternatives listed in the recipe.

Recipe: See page 198.

Bodily Consumption: 64 ounces per day between each meal and snack, in Green Life Cocktail, and in frappés.

Spiced Lemon Toddy

Benefits: D-limonine antioxidant helps the liver break down fat-trapping toxins and thins bile. A pinch of fragrant cinnamon and ginger will give your metabolism an added boost.

Brands: For ginger and cinnamon: Frontier Herbs, Simply Organic, and The Spice Hunter

Recipe: See page 200.

Bodily Consumption: Daily on arising

Green Life Cocktail

Benefits: High in chlorophyll content, which helps to detoxify organs, especially the liver. Purifies the blood, is rich in vitamin K (necessary for blood clotting), and is the basis of "blood" for plants. Helps build red blood cells to carry oxygen to every cell of your body.

Brands: Pure powdered wheat grass or UNI KEY's Liver-Lovin' Formula

Recipe: See page 199.

Bodily Consumption: Daily on arising

Probiotic Sweetener

Benefits: Contains beneficial bacteria to balance GI tract for weight-loss insurance and enhanced immunity. Provides yeast-free sweetener for no-heat frappés, beverages, and desserts.

Brand: UNI KEY's Flora-Key

Bodily Consumption: 2 to 3 teaspoons per day in Green Life Cocktails, frappés, and in nonheated foods

Whey Protein

Benefits: Assists lean muscle mass development, increases energy, natural appetite suppressant

Brands: UNI KEY's Fat Flush Vanilla or Chocolate Whey Protein

Bodily Consumption: Up to 2 servings per day (20 grams protein each) in frappés, muffins, desserts, whey pancakes, etc. Note: Chocolate whey is limited to 2 servings per week.

Chia Seeds

Benefits: Great source of omega-3 and plant-based calcium plus a major hunger buster due to high fiber content. Also bulks up stools, which help rid your intestines of toxic buildup.

Brand: Omega3 Chia Seeds

Bodily Consumption: 2 to 3 tablespoons per day, added to frappés, soups, stews, and dressings, or sprinkled on foods such as eggs and veggies

Slimming Oils
Choose from:
High-Lignan Flaxseed Oil
Benefits: Natural anti-inflammatory that inhibits weight gain; helps keep blood sugar levels even, provides satiety and balanced hormones. A good source for omega-3 fatty acids.
Brands: Omega Nutrition, Health from the Sun, and Spectrum
Bodily Consumption: Total of 1 tablespoon per day of either flaxseed oil or fish oil. Do not heat flaxseed oil.

Fish Oil
Benefits: High in EPA and DHA; provides increased oxidation of fat cells; reduces inflammation; boosts brain, joint, and cardiovascular health
Brands: Brands with fish oil products that are molecularly distilled and contaminant-free via third-party testings.
Bodily Consumption: Total of 1 tablespoon per day of either flaxseed oil or fish oil. Do not heat fish oil.

Add another tablespoon of one of the following in addition to the flaxseed oil and/or fish oil:

Extra-Virgin Olive Oil
Benefits: Provides antibacterial benefits, aids the heart, and reduces inflammation; natural painkiller.
Brands: Spectrum, Bionaturae, Newman's Own, Bertolli, Lucini, Spectrm in an oil mister (such as Misto)

Macadamia Nut Oil
Benefits: Oil highest in MUFAs; increases omega-3s into cell membranes and raises HDL for overall health.
Brand: MacNut Oil

Coconut Oil
Benefits: Anti-*Candida* and antifungal; supports healthy gut ecology; aids weight loss by providing medium-chain triglycerides that are used as fuel
Brands: Nutiva Extra-Virgin

Sesame Oil

Benefits: Enhances the liver's ability to burn fat and is high in the antioxidant sesamol, which maintains stability under high temperatures.

Brands: Spectrum, Eden

Herbs, Spices, and Seasonings

Benefits: Enticing flavor enhancers provide digestive power, act as a natural phyto-estrogen, and are aromatic and warming to the soul. They are also natural diuretics, anti-inflammatories, and heavy metal chelators.

Brands: Nonirradiated herbs and spices from Frontier Herbs, Simply Organic, and the Spice Hunter

Choose from:

Allspice

Anise   Fennel (fresh or dried)

Apple cider vinegar   Garlic (fresh or garlic powder)

Basil (fresh or dried)   Ginger (fresh or dried)

Bay leaves (fresh or dried)   Horseradish

Caraway seeds   Marjoram (fresh or dried)

Cardamom   Nutmeg

Cayenne   Onion powder

Chinese five-spice powder   Oregano (fresh or dried)

Chives (fresh or dried)   Parsley (fresh or dried)

Cilantro   Poppy seeds

Cinnamon   Rosemary (fresh or dried)

Cloves   Saffron

Coriander   Sage (fresh or dried)

Cream of tartar   Savory (fresh or dried)

Cumin   Tarragon (fresh or dried)

Dijon mustard (without added sugar)   Thyme (fresh or dried)

Dill (fresh or dried)   Turmeric

Dry mustard   Wasabi

Bodily Consumption: ¼ to ½ teaspoon at least 3 to 5 times per week

Protein

Benefits: Activates the liver's detox enzymes, raises your metabolism by nearly 30 percent, and produces glucagon to balance insulin.

Brands: See below

Bodily Consumption: A minimum of 8 ounces of cooked lean protein

Choose from:

Suggested varieties of canned or fresh fish, shellfish and seafood (wild encouraged)

Lean beef, lamb, veal (organic/grass-fed encouraged), and other meats

Poultry, hormone-free and free-range preferred

Omega-enriched eggs (hormone-free/free-range encouraged)

Vegetarian Protein Sources: Tofu and tempeh

Fish

Choose from:

Fresh
- Bass
- Cod
- Grouper
- Haddock
- Halibut
- Mackerel
- Mahimahi
- Orange roughy
- Perch
- Pike
- Pollock
- Salmon
- Sardines
- Snapper
- Sole
- Squid
- Trout
- Tuna
- Whitefish

Canned
- Crabmeat (Featherweight, Seasons, Lillie, Three Star)
- Light tuna—not albacore (Natural Sea, Crown Prince)
- Mackerel

Salmon (Natural Sea, Crown Prince, Vital Choice)

Sardines (Bela, Olhao, Crown Prince)

Shellfish
- Calamari
- Crab
- Lobster
- Scallops
- Shrimp

Meat

Choose from: Lean beef, lamb, veal, and other meats

Look for free-range, grass-fed lean meat found in health food stores or supermarkets or online companies such as Niman Ranch (www.nimanranch.com). My personal favorite is Ranch Foods Direct (www.ranchfoodsdirect.com), a specialty meat company selling natural beef, raised without hormones or antibiotics. This company combines the best of traditional animal husbandry practices with an innovative processing method.

Beef	*Lamb*	*Other Meats*
Brisket	Leg	Elk
Chuck	Loin	Ostrich
Eye of round	Rib	Venison
Flank	*Veal*	Bison from Hole
London broil	Loin	Buffalo Company
Round	Rib	(www.jhbuffalomeat
Rump	Shoulder	.com) and Buffalo Gal
Sirloin		(www.buffalogal.com)

Poultry
Choose from:
White meat of skinned turkey and chicken, fresh or frozen. Look for free-range and hormone-free, such as Foster Farms, Harmony Farms, Shelton Farms, and Young Farms.

In addition to the above protein choices you may also enjoy:

Omega-Enriched Eggs
Benefits: Highest-quality protein on the planet; contains sulfur-bearing aminos that help detox process, brain nutrients, and superstar antioxidants lutein and zeanxathine that maintain eyes.
Brands: Organic Valley, Gold Circle Farms, Country Hen, Eggland's Best, Pilgrim's Pride Eggs Plus
Bodily Consumption: Up to 2 per day

Vegetarian Protein Sources
Choose from:
Tofu—unflavored, firm and silken (Mori-Nu, White Wave)
Tempeh (Turtle Island Foods, Lightlife)
Bodily Consumption: Up to 2 servings (4 ounces each) of tofu and/or tempeh per week

Fruits
Benefits: The following healthy fruits offer collagen-enhancing vitamin C and enzyme-activating potassium, and they help maintain balanced blood sugar.
Brands (frozen): Frozen fruits are acceptable as well, such as Woodstock Farms (www.woodstock-farms.com), Cascadian Farm (www.cfarm.com), and Stahlbush Farm (www.stahlbush.com).
Bodily Consumption: Up to 2 servings per day

Choose from:

1 small apple, orange, nectarine, peach, pear, or pomegranate

½ cup organic plain or raspberry applesauce (Solana Gold)

1 cup berries (blueberries, blackberries, raspberries, and/or cranberries)

6 large strawberries

10 large cherries

2 medium-size plums

½ grapefruit

Lemons and limes (as desired)

Vegetables

Benefits: Full of sweeping fiber, the following low-glycemic and carotenoid-rich veggies speed up the liver's cleansing process and offer enzymes, vital minerals, and chlorophyll for radiant health and good looks.

Fresh: Look for fresh (in season locally is best) vegetables that are full of vibrant color so that you can eat the rainbow.

Brands (frozen): Frozen vegetables are acceptable as well, such as Woodstock Farms (www.woodstock-farms.com), Cascadian Farm (www.cfarm.com), and Stahlbush Farm (www.stahlbush.com).

Brands (canned): No added salt or sugar

Bodily Consumption: Aim for at least 5 or more servings per day. A vegetable serving is generally 1 cup raw or ½ cup cooked.

Choose from:

(All unlimited except where noted)

Artichokes (1 whole or 5 hearts)

Arugula

Asparagus

Bamboo shoots

Bell peppers (red, green, and orange)

Bok choy

Broccoli

Brussels sprouts

Burdock

Cabbage

Carrots (limit 1 medium-size or 5 baby)

Cauliflower

Celery

Celery root

Chard

Chinese cabbage

Chives

Cilantro

Collard greens

Cucumbers

Daikon

Dandelion greens

Eggplant

Endive

Escarole

Green beans

Hearts of palm

Jalapeños

Jerusalem artichoke

Jicama

Kale

Kohlrabi

Leeks

Lettuce (red or green, romaine, butter, baby greens, etc.)

Mushrooms

Mustard greens

Okra

Olives (black, 3 per day)

Onions

Parsley

Radicchio

Radishes

Rhubarb (1 cup)	tomato products (see	Diced tomatoes
Shallots	below)	Pizza sauce
Snow peas	Water chestnuts	Tomato paste
Spaghetti squash	Watercress	Tomato puree
Spinach	Yellow squash	Tomato sauce
Sprouts (alfalfa,	Zucchini	Whole peeled
mung bean, broccoli)		tomatoes
Sugar snap peas	*Tomato Products* (no	*Brands:* Muir Glen,
Tomatillos	added sugar or	Eden, Bio Nature,
Tomatoes and	salt)	Woodstock Farms

Sea Vegetables

Benefits: Rich in iodine and many trace minerals such as calcium and iron, sea veggies support thyroid function and also inhibit the absorption of radiation and heavy metals.

Choose from: Agar, arame, hijiki, kombu, nori, sea palm fronds, wakame

Brand: Eden

Bodily Consumption: Up to 2 servings of 1 tablespoon agar and/or ½ cup of arame, hijiki, kombu, nori, sea palm fronds, and wakame per week added to soups, stews, poultry, beef, fish, seafood, salads, veggies, eggs, etc.

You may also add a sea veggie–based seasoning:

Brand: Eden Seaweed Gomasio (contains sea vegetables, sesame seeds, and sea salt)

Bodily Consumption: ½ teaspoon daily

CLEAN CARBS

In Winter Fat Flush, warming Clean Carbs are part of the menu plan, but you'll consume them sparingly and choose from a list of Clean Carbs that are divided into four sections: starchy vegetables; tortillas, crackers, and chips; gluten-free cereals and grains; and legumes. In Month 1, many dieters find they do best with just one or two starchy vegetables or one starchy veggie and one slice of bread or tortilla per day. In Month 2, add a third Clean Carb from any of the remaining categories. When you reach Month 3, you may consume a total of three to four Clean Carbs per day from any category to provide warmth and satisfaction on those cold winter days. If you feel bloated, tired, or experience cravings (classic signs of food sensitivities) with any of these additional choices, then cut out the suspect Clean Carb until your symptoms are gone or you choose another selection that may be more in tune with your body.

Starchy Vegetables (cooked)

Benefits: Rated moderately low on the glycemic index, these nutrient-dense, slow-acting, rainbow-colored carbs provide additional "smart" calories to help fuel workouts and promote a feeling of fullness. Traditional Chinese medicine views root veggies (like parsnips, turnips, and rutabagas) as warming foods that aid digestion and help cleanse the liver.

Choose from:

1 small sweet potato or yam
½ cup green peas
½ cup carrots
½ cup winter squash (such as butternut, Delicata, hubbard, acorn, and kabocha)
½ cup parsnips

½ cup pumpkin (fresh or unsweetened pure canned)
½ cup turnips
½ cup rutabagas
½ cup beets (red and golden)
½ cup corn
½ cup potatoes, or 1 small baked

Bread and Tortillas

Benefits: Gut-friendly flours full of fiber and easy on digestion. Sprouted grains also benefit, the GI tract with maximized mineral, vitamin, and enzyme content for better digestion and utilization.

Brands: French Meadow Healthseed Spelt Bread (yeast-free); Kinnikinnick Candadi Multigrain Rice Bread (yeast- and gluten-free); Food for Life Ezekiel 4:9 Sprouted Whole Grain Tortilla (yeast- and gluten-free); Food for Life Sprouted Corn Tortilla (yeast- and gluten-free)

Bodily Consumption: 1 slice bread or 1 (6-inch) tortilla

Grains and Cereals

Quinoa

Benefit: The "Mother of All Grains" is the highest in amino acids of grains—although technically it is a seed.

Brands: Bob's Red Mill, Ancient Harvest

Bodily Consumption: ½ cup cooked

Oatmeal (rolled or steel-cut)

Benefit: High source of beta-glucan that can lower cholesterol

Brands: Quaker, Bob's Red Mill

Bodily Consumption: ½ cup cooked

Other Cereals and Grains

Choose from:

½ cup brown or wild rice, cooked (Lundberg Family Farms)

½ cup whole-grain pasta, cooked (Hodgson Mill)

½ cup spelt or rice pasta, cooked (Tinkyada, Eden)

½ cup toasted buckwheat or amaranth cereal, cooked

3 cups plain popcorn (popped)

Crackers and Chips
Choose from:

2 Scandinavian-style crispbreads
   (Wasa, Kauli, Bran-a-Crisp)

5 brown rice crackers

7 blue corn chips (Garden of Eatin)

Legumes (cooked)
Choose from:

½ cup red or green lentils

½ cup black, pinto, or garbanzo beans
   (chickpeas)

½ cup yellow or green split peas

Brands (canned): Eden with kombu,
   Westbrae

Dairy
For Month 1, include one serving per day from any of the lists below. In Months 2 and
   3, you may include (if you like) up to two servings (total) of dairy per day.

Benefits: These calcium-rich foods provide added variety to meals, snacks, and recipes.

Cheese (hard and semisoft)
Choose from:

Cheddar

Feta

Goat

Mozzarella

Parmesan

Romano

String

Swiss

Brands: Horizon, Organic Valley

Bodily Consumption: 1 ounce

Cottage and Ricotta Cheese
Brands: Friendship, Old House

Bodily Consumption: ½ cup

Yogurt (plain nonfat, low-fat, or whole milk)
Brands: Fage (Greek), Nancy's, Stonyfield,
   Cascade, Horizon, Brown Cow

Bodily Consumption: 1 cup

Kefir (plain)
Brand: Lifeway

Bodily Consumption: 1 cup

Nuts, Seeds, Nut Butters, and Friendly Fats
Choose from:

7 almonds or filberts

3 macadamia nuts

4 pecan or walnut halves

4 large chestnuts

1 tablespoon seeds (sesame, pumpkin,
   and/or sunflower)

1 tablespoon almond, peanut, and/or
   sesame-tahini butter (Westbrae,
   Arrowhead Mills, Maranatha)

½ small avocado

1 tablespoon of cream cheese

1 tablespoon sour cream

1 pat of butter
1 tablespoon unsweetened coconut

Beverages (optional)

Vegetable Juices

Benefits: High in antioxidants and vitamins; adds variety to beverage choices

Brands: V8 Juice, Knudsen Organic Very Veggie Juice

Bodily Consumption: 8 ounces per day

Legal Cheats

Turkey Bacon

Brand: Applegate Farms

Bodily Consumption: 1 to 2 slices per day

Alcohol (grain-free)

Choose from:

Potato vodka

Rum (made from sugar)

Tequila (from the cactus plant)

Bodily Consumption: 1 ounce mixed with water, Cranberry H_2O, or unflavored sparkling water once a week

Sparkling Water (unflavored)

Brands: Perrier, San Pellegrino

Bodily Consumption: 8 ounces, 2 to 3 times per week

Organic Coffee—caffeinated

Benefits: Provides antioxidants and B vitamins such as niacin

Brands: Newman's Own Organics, Organic Coffee Co.

Bodily Consumption: 1 cup per day

Bodily Consumption: 1 serving per day

Healing Tea

Nettle

Benefit: Rich in alkalizing minerals, which aid kidney cleansing

Brands: Alvita, Traditional Medicinals

Bodily Consumption: 1 to 2 cups per day

Cocoa Powder

Benefits: High in antioxidant (flavonoids) and magnesium, which relaxes system

Brands: Green & Black, Hershey's

Bodily Consumption: 1 teaspoon once a week

Carob Powder

Benefit: Mineral-rich substitute for those reactive to cocoa

Brands: Frontier

Bodily Consumption: 1 teaspoon once a week

Cacao Powder

Benefit: Food highest in polyphenols (type of antioxidant)

Brands: Sunfood Nutrition, TerrAmazon

Bodily Consumption: 1 teaspoon once a week

Flavor Extracts

Benefit: Provides flavor enhancer without added carbs or fats

Brands: Frontier, Simply Organic, Nature's Flavors

Choose from:

Anise

Almond

Lemon

Mint

Orange

Rum

Vanilla

Bodily Consumption: ¼ to ½ teaspoon as needed

Salt

Benefits: Aids digestion and acid/alkaline balance

Brands: Morton's Canning and Pickling Salt, Real Salt, Himalayan Pink Salt

Bodily Consumption: ½ to 1 teaspoon per day. (Use your best judgment—if you bloat, are hypertensive, or take a diuretic, take less. If you have low blood pressure or suffer from adrenal exhaustion, you can use up to 1 teaspoon per day.)

Stevia Plus (for use in heated foods)

Bodily Consumption: Maximum of 2 (0.035-ounce or 1-gram) packets per day

A GENTLE REMINDER—ESPECIALLY FOR WINTER FAT FLUSH

■ Menu plans are completely optional. If following a structured plan is not for you, feel free to create your own fabulous Fat Flush–friendly meals and snacks that follow the Winter Fat Flush guidelines.

■ Recipes noted with an asterisk (*) are found in chapter 21.

■ Lunches and dinners are interchangeable within the same day.

■ You may add an extra tablespoon of chia seeds into recipes, if desired.

■ Make sure to drink a total of 64 ounces of Cranberry H_2O, heated just enough to take out the chill, daily between meals. Eight ounces of Cranberry H_2O are included in a daily Green Life Cocktail. You may drink as much plain filtered water as you like. You may also enjoy a cup of organic coffee and a cup or two of nettle tea per day. Two to three times a week, you may have a glass of sparkling water.

■ Optimize your results with the Fat Flush Kit supplements: the Dieters' Multi (with or without iron) for balanced vitamin and mineral supplementation; the GLA 90s for stimulating brown adipose tissue metabolism that increases fat burning, and the Weight-Loss Formula for carbohydrate control, fat metabolism, and liver support (without stimulants).

■ Take 1,000 mg of CLA (conjugated linolenic acid) with each meal to help retain lean muscle mass, protect against heart disease, and modulate the immune response. You'll continue to take this throughout the program.

WINTER FAT FLUSH: 7-DAY MEAL PLANNER (MONTH 1)

DAY 1

On Arising
  Spiced Lemon Toddy* (page 200)
  Green Life Cocktail* (page199)

Breakfast
  Sunshine Frittata* (page 206) with 1 table-
    spoon of chia seeds
  1 slice French Meadow Healthseed Spelt
    Bread, toasted, drizzled with 1 table-
    spoon of flaxseed oil
  1 orange

Snack
  ½ cup ricotta cheese with 1 teaspoon of
    Flora-Key and 1 tablespoon toasted
    pumpkin seeds

Lunch
  1 cup Curried Delicata Squash Bisque*
    (page 233)
  4 ounces sardines, plus red onion and
    broccoli sprouts wrapped in large let-
    tuce leaves with Dijon mustard

Snack
  Pears 'n' Cinnamon Frappé* (page 202)

Dinner
  4 ounces roast turkey with marjoram and
    lemon
  Pan-seared cauliflower, broccoli, and Brus-
    sels sprouts with lemon

  Timesaver Tip! *Save 4 ounces turkey for Day
  3's Lunch.*

DAY 2

On Arising
  Spiced Lemon Toddy* (page 200)
  Green Life Cocktail* (page 199)

Breakfast
  Raspberry Truffle Frappé* (page 202)
  1 poached egg

Snack
  Artichoke, Olive, and Goat Cheese Piz-
    zetta made with 1 Ezekiel 4:9 tortilla,
    3 chopped artichoke hearts, 3 sliced
    black olives, 1 ounce of goat cheese,
    and 1 tablespoon of chopped fresh
    parsley. Bake at 425°F for 5 minutes, or
    until the cheese is bubbly.

Lunch
  Salmon Salad on bed of baby greens,
    made with 4 ounces of canned salmon,
    plus seeded and chopped red pepper,
    celery, 1 sliced hard-boiled egg, and
    2 tablespoons of Herbal Dijon Vinai-
    grette* (page 238)

Snack
  1 pear and 7 almonds

Dinner
  4 ounces grilled veal chop rubbed with
    Garam Masala*
  ½ cup corn sprinkled with Seaweed
    Gomasio
  Steamed broccoli rabe with thyme

DAY 3

On Arising
Spiced Lemon Toddy* (page 200)
Green Life Cocktail* (page 199)

Breakfast
2 scrambled eggs with pinch of tarragon
1 slice French Meadow Healthseed Spelt
   Bread, toasted, with 1 tablespoon of
   cream cheese

Snack
Berries 'n' Cherries Frappé* (page 202)

Lunch
4 ounces leftover roast turkey
Steamed chard with ground coriander and
   1 tablespoon of olive oil

Snack
1 apple
1 Fabulous Chia Crax* (page246)
1 ounce cheddar cheese

Dinner
4 ounces grilled beef burger with Dijon
   mustard
1 small baked potato with chopped fresh
   dill
Grilled eggplant slices

Fat Flush on the Fly: *Applegate Farms 100%
Organic Beef*

Timesaver Tip! *Save a beef burger for Day 4's
Lunch.*

DAY 4

On Arising
Spiced Lemon Toddy* (page 200)
Green Life Cocktail* (page 199)

Breakfast
Peachy Keene Frappé* (page 203)

Snack
1 Fabulous Chia Crax* (page 246)
Zucchini and yellow squash rounds (raw)

Lunch
Beef Burger Burrito made with 1 leftover
   beef burger, chopped tomatoes, bell
   pepper, red onion, and 1 tablespoon
   of salsa wrapped in 1 warmed Ezekiel
   4:9 tortilla

Snack
2 hard-boiled eggs
½ grapefruit

Fat Flush on the Fly: *Eggland's Best Hard-
Cooked Peeled Eggs*

Dinner
4 ounces roasted leg of lamb rubbed with
   Fat Flush Seasoning* (page 235)
½ cup roasted beets with chopped fresh
   parsley
Steamed broccoli and cauliflower with
   marjoram and 1 tablespoon of
   flaxseed oil

Timesaver Tip! *Save 4 ounces leg of lamb for
Day 5's Lunch.*

DAY 5

On Arising
Spiced Lemon Toddy* (page 200)
Green Life Cocktail* (page 199)

Breakfast
2 poached eggs on a bed of steamed
fennel
1 slice French Meadow Healthseed Spelt
Bread, toasted

Snack
½ cup applesauce
1 tablespoon toasted sunflower seeds

Lunch
Dragon Bowl Salad* (page 219) made with
4 ounces leftover leg of lamb and 2
tablespoons Herbal Dijon Vinaigrette*
(page 238)

Snack
1 Fabulous Chia Crax* (page 246) sprinkled
with 1 teaspoon of Flora-Key

Dinner
1 serving Pan-Seared Shrimp with Fresh
Corn Salsa* (page 218)
Roasted green beans with garlic and basil

Dessert
Black 'n White Yogurt Parfait* (page 241)

DAY 6

On Arising
Spiced Lemon Toddy* (page 200)
Green Life Cocktail* (page 199)

Breakfast
Rhubarb-Berry Burst Frappé* (page 202)
2 scrambled eggs with marjoram and
thyme

Snack
Chopped veggies and 1 ounce of Swiss
cheese melted on an Ezekiel 4:9 tortilla

Lunch
2 cups 'Shrooms 'n' Tempeh Chili* (page
222) sprinkled with toasted nori
crumbles (toasted nori crumbles are
made with 1 sheet of nori, toasted and
crumbled).

Snack
½ cup raspberry applesauce
1 Fabulous Chia Crax* (page 246)

Dinner
1 serving Tilapia with Spinach-Walnut Pesto* (page 218)
Oven-roasted artichoke halves sprinkled
with thyme
½ cup steamed baby new potatoes with 1
teaspoon of caraway seeds

DAY 7

On Arising
Spiced Lemon Toddy* (page 200)
Green Life Cocktail* (page 199)

Breakfast
Egg and Turkey Bacon Burrito* (page 207)

Snack
1 Fabulous Chia Crax* (page 246) with
    1 tablespoon of almond butter
Orange, red, and yellow bell pepper rings

Lunch
Confetti Salad with Tuna made with 4
    ounces of canned tuna, 1 chopped
    hard-boiled egg, and ½ cup each grat-
    ed raw beets, zucchini, and jicama, with
    2 tablespoons of Mediterranean Vinai-
    grette* (page 238)

Snack
Blueberry Heaven Frappé* (page 203)

Dinner
1 serving Persian Meatball and Vegetable
    Skewers* (page 218)
Steamed spaghetti squash with ground
    coriander and allspice

Dessert
1 cup blackberries tossed with 1 teaspoon
    of Flora-Key

WINTER FAT FLUSH: 7-DAY MEAL PLANNER (MONTH 3)

DAY 1

On Arising
Spiced Lemon Toddy* (page 200)
Green Life Cocktail* (page 199)

Breakfast
Choco-Rhuberry Frappé* (page 202)
2 slices French Meadow Healthseed Spelt
    Bread, toasted

Snack
Celery and jicama sticks with 2 table-
    spoons of salsa
1 hard-boiled egg

Lunch
Romaine salad with grape tomatoes and
    hearts of palm
4 ounces canned salmon, 1 sliced hard-
    boiled egg, and 1 tablespoon of
    lemon-flavored fish oil
7 blue corn chips

Fat Flush on the Fly: *Eggland's Best Hard-
    Cooked Peeled Eggs*

Snack
2 plums and 1 ounce Swiss cheese

Dinner
2 cups Chicken Cacciatore* (page 210)
Steamed cauliflower mashed with marjo-
    ram and 1 tablespoon of chia seeds
½ cup oven-roasted baby red potatoes
    with ground coriander

Timesaver Tip! *Save extra Chicken Cacciatore
    for Day 4's Lunch.*

DAY 2

On Arising
Spiced Lemon Toddy* (page 200)
Green Life Cocktail* (page 199)

Breakfast
1 serving Break of Dawn Oatmeal* (page 205) with 1 tablespoon of chia seeds
1 soft-boiled egg with pinch of Seaweed Gomasio

Snack
½ cup ricotta cheese mixed with ground nutmeg and 1 teaspoon of Flora-Key

Lunch
Dragon Bowl Salad (page 219) topped with 4 ounces of canned tuna, 1 tablespoon of toasted sesame seeds, 1 chopped hard-boiled egg, and 2 tablespoons of Sesame Vinaigrette* (page 238)
1 Ezekiel 4:9 tortilla

Fat Flush on the Fly: *Bragg Sesame & Ginger Salad Dressing*

Snack
Pears 'n' Cinnamon Frappé* (page 202)

Dinner
4 ounces grilled sirloin with Fat Flush Seasoning* (page 235)
Steamed sugar snap peas with thyme and 1 tablespoon of flaxseed oil
½ cup steamed rutabaga with dill

Timesaver Tip! *Grill an extra 4-ounce sirloin for Day 3's Lunch.*

DAY 3

On Arising
Spiced Lemon Toddy* (page 200)
Green Life Cocktail* (page 199)

Breakfast
Wild Berry Crunch Frappé* (page 203)

Snack
Roasted Red Pepper and Fresh Mozzarella Flatbread made with 1 Ezekiel 4:9 tortilla, roasted red peppers, 1 ounce of fresh mozzarella cheese, and fresh basil. Bake at 425°F for 5 minutes, or until the cheese is bubbly.

Lunch
Baby greens salad with cucumbers, tomatoes, 3 olives, and 4 ounces of leftover sirloin

2 tablespoons Herbal Dijon Vinaigrette* (page 238)
2 Scandinavian-style crispbreads

Snack
2 hard-boiled eggs with 2 tablespoons of salsa

Dinner
4 ounces grilled mahimahi
½ cup oven-roasted butternut squash with 1 tablespoon of chia seeds and pinch of Seaweed Gomasio
Steamed Broccoflower or broccoli with lemon and 1 teaspoon of caraway seeds

Dessert
1 cup Ginger Peach Sorbet* (page 239)

DAY 4

On Arising
Spiced Lemon Toddy* (page 200)
Green Life Cocktail* (page 199)

Breakfast
2 poached eggs over steamed chard with
    pinch of Seaweed Gomasio and 1
    tablespoon of chia seeds
1 slice French Meadow Healthseed Spelt
    Bread, toasted
1 tablespoon of cream cheese

Snack
1 apple and 1 ounce of Swiss cheese

Lunch
2 cups leftover Chicken Cacciatore* with ½
    cup of cooked whole-grain pasta
Steamed kale with garlic and 1 tablespoon
    of freshly squeezed lime juice

Snack
Peanut Butter Sundae Frappé* (page 203)

Dinner
2 cups Beet Borscht* (page 233)
4 ounces broiled lamb burger with Dijon
    mustard
Pan-seared asparagus with tarragon and 1
    tablespoon of olive oil

Fat Flush on the Fly: *In a hurry for dinner?
Try Imagine's Organic Potato Leek Soup
instead of the borscht.*

Timesaver Tip! *Save leftover soup and broil
an extra lamb patty for Day 5's Lunch.*

DAY 5

On Arising
Spiced Lemon Toddy* (page 200)
Green Life Cocktail* (page 199)

Breakfast
Raspberry Rapture Frappé* (page 203)

Snack
½ cup avocado mashed with 1 tablespoon
    of freshly squeezed lime juice and
    cayenne·
1 corn tortilla, cut into wedges and toasted

Lunch
2 cups leftover Beet Borscht*
4 ounces leftover lamb burger
Sliced cucumbers with chopped fresh dill

Snack
½ cup applesauce
2 hard-boiled eggs

Dinner
1 serving Soft Tacos Olé * (page 213)
½ cup steamed snow peas with lemon and
    1 tablespoon of chia seeds
Wilted red cabbage salad with cilantro and
    1 tablespoon each of freshly squeezed
    lime juice and flaxseed oil

DAY 6

On Arising
Spiced Lemon Toddy* (page 200)
Green Life Cocktail* (page 199)

Breakfast
2 eggs scrambled with orange and red peppers and marjoram
½ cup toasted buckwheat with ground cinnamon and 4 toasted chopped walnut halves

Snack
½ cup cottage cheese with 1 small pear

Lunch
1 serving Asian Arame Salad* (page 220)
1 slice French Meadow Healthseed Spelt Bread, toasted

Snack
Strawberry Cream Frappé* (page 202)

Dinner
4 ounces grilled scallops with Fat Flush Seasoning* (page 235)
½ cup oven-roasted acorn squash with pinch of ground ginger
Steamed mixed greens (such as kale, chard, and mustard) with lemon juice and 1 tablespoon of chia seeds

DAY 7

On Arising
Spiced Lemon Toddy* (page 200)
Green Life Cocktail* (page 199)

Breakfast
Blueberry Mini Chiacakes* (page 204)

Snack
1 ounce cheddar cheese
1 hard-boiled egg
1 tablespoon toasted pumpkin seeds

Lunch
Dragon Bowl Salad* (page 219) made with 4 ounces of shrimp and 2 tablespoons of Mediterranean Vinaigrette* (page 238)
7 blue corn chips

Fat Flush on the Fly: *Use precooked fresh or frozen peeled and deveined shrimp.*

Snack
½ cup Chickpea Tahini Pâté* (page 249)
Snow pea and endive dippers
1 Ezekiel 4:9 tortilla

Dinner
4 ounces Roasted Moroccan Spiced Chicken* (page 209)
½ cup pan-roasted carrots with ground cardamom
Steamed broccolini with 1 tablespoon of lemon-flavored fish oil

Dessert
Baked apple topped with ground allspice, 1 tablespoon of chia seeds, and 1 teaspoon of Flora-Key

9 WINTER WELLNESS PROGRAM

WINTER IS THE IDEAL TIME TO DO A BASELINE, overall blood test assessment. Your doctor can order a comprehensive blood panel that will measure a variety of basic health indicators, including a complete blood count, lipid profiles, and glucose levels, as well your liver enzymes.

For Fat Flushing purposes, assessing your liver can be a lifesaving step. Unlike the heart or the lungs, where you get clear-cut signs that something is amiss (such as a racing heart, angina, arrhythmia, or difficulty breathing), your liver doesn't let you know that there is a problem until it's too late. I want to make sure that your liver, and its sister organ, the gallbladder, are functioning properly and breaking down fats so that weight loss and your overall health are not impeded. Do make sure that the overall blood test includes the liver enzyme tests GGTP (gallbladder/bile enzyme test) and SGOT (hepatitis, chemical poisoning, cirrhosis test).

A score above the normal lab reference range can suggest a damaged or inflamed liver and/or gallbladder. Fat Flushing, in general, will support both of these organs. Many Fat Flushers have found that their liver enzymes are normalized by the program. A liver-supporting dietary supplement formula that includes milk thistle extract, Oregon grape root, dandelion, and alpha lipoic acid helps ensure that these organs are working efficiently. In any case, consult with your physician.

Keep in mind that if your liver is not functioning properly, you will not be able to break down hormones, whether they are "natural" or synthetic, which can be an underlying factor in bloating, weight gain, and water retention. So, once you have determined that all of your liver function tests are in line, I recommend a salivary hormone test, which you will be introduced to in Summer Fat Flush.

This is also a good time to get your vitamin D levels assessed, so make sure to ask your doctor to order this special test in addition to the blood panel. Getting enough vitamin D is important for your overall health to protect against colds, influenza, and other infections. It may also help protect against diabetes, hypertension, heart disease, and certain cancers.[1]

> ## Healing Winter Rituals
>
> Set aside one day each week to rest, reflect, and regenerate (Sabbath ritual).
> Meditate for at least 10 minutes a day to deeply rest your mind.

Vitamin D expert John Cannell, MD, believes that vitamin D levels should optimally be between 50 to 70 ng/ml year round. I recommend you take between 4,000 and 5,000 IUs during the winter and at least 1,000 to 2,000 IUs in the summer. Be sure to take the natural form of this nutrient, which is D_3.

WINTER BACH FLOWER REMEDY

You were introduced to the Bach Flower Remedies in Pre–Fat Flush Wellness and I trust you've already begun to experience the difference they can make: renewed energy, a can-do spirit, and a revitalized inner well-being. Now you will again benefit from flower power. The Bach Flower Remedy Oak will enhance your will power, endurance, and your devotion to higher ideals. As you did before, add four drops to eight ounces of plain water or Cranberry H_2O four times a day, dab it on your skin, or put a few drops in your bath.

YOU KNOW YOU ARE A FAT FLUSHER WHEN... you start making to-do lists and actually do them.

> *This Saturday will be six weeks that I've been Fat Flushing and I am feeling like a new man. Thinking more lucidly, body is moving more fluidly, just a great turnaround. I was feeling so depressed before I started this…and now with the almost six weeks of no sugar, I'm so happy to report that the mind is alert and alive and not depressed.*
>
> *—Stephen, Fat Flush Fan*

ADVANCED WINTER DETOX TECHNIQUES

My years of experience with cutting-edge detox has convinced me that to achieve and maintain weight loss and optimal health, you need to integrate into your program more advanced detox techniques that go beyond diet and exercise. Winter Wellness offers advanced techniques that will sustain you through every season for the rest of your life. Taking advantage of these methods is a great way to free your body from the myriad toxins that fill our modern world. Nobody is immune, including newborns, to the thousands of pesticides, solvents, and drugs in our environment these days. (Nearly two hundred industrial chemicals are found in the umbilical cord blood of babies—a shocking statistic.) Lingering saboteurs can not only stall your weight loss but sap your health and vitality.

Dry Heat Sauna (start with 5 minutes and work up to 20, 2 to 3 times per week)

Sweat is much more than a body temperature regulator. It helps to detoxify the body of heavy metals and nasty fat-storage toxins. Remember that the skin is your largest external organ and helps to relieve the toxic overload on the liver and kidneys. Most people lose up to a quart of water through plain sweating. But, if you are in a sauna, you'll release that quart of water in just fifteen minutes. So this is why sauna therapy is the perfect way to lessen your body's toxic load.

Sweating is not just a good detox, it's also good for your heart and your body. Blood flow is improved while your heart gets a very gentle workout. Besides cardiovascular benefits, sauna therapy can help musculoskeletal pain, arthritis, chronic fatigue, and depression.

For a list of my recommended home saunas, see resources, page 263. If a home sauna is not in your budget, try to work out a deal with a local hotel or fitness centers that have saunas. Oftentimes you can pay a nominal fee for access to their equipment.

> ### Rejuvenating Winter Mini-Indulgences
>
> Treat yourself to a spa, cruise, or vacation in a warmer climate.
> Pamper yourself with a hot stone treatment and warming herbal wraps.

Oil Pulling (20 minutes, upon rising before you eat)

Oil pulling is a simple yet highly beneficial method of cleansing your mouth as well as detoxing your entire system. Your mouth is the repository of a tremendous amount of bacteria that can impact different areas of your body. Dentists who practice holistic and biological dentistry believe that each tooth is connected to an organ. If that tooth has a root canal, is decayed (even under a crown that X-rays don't pick up), is an implant, or even has been pulled, leaving behind a cavitation (hole in the jawbone), you can experience a whole host of health challenges in the associated meridian line of that tooth. This means that your unresolved digestive problem (teeth 2, 3, 28, 29), irritable bowel syndrome (tooth 6), or even liver dysfunction (teeth 11 and 12) may be associated with the anaerobic bacteria seeping into your system from root canals, implants, and cavitations affecting these teeth. This can dramatically impact your system, making you ill in varying degrees. To get an idea of how your mouth affects your total physical and emotional well-being (and illness), check out the chart on page 87.

It Really Is All in Your Head

As you can see, it is very important to clean up and detoxify the "hidden" bacteria in your teeth and gums. The tricky thing is that most of these bacteria are hidden

Acumeridian Tooth-Organ Relationships
[with Autonomic/Neuropeptide Emotion correlations]

Upper Teeth

Tooth #	Organ	Sinus / Body Correlations	Emotions
1	Heart, Small Int., Circulation/Sex, Endocrine	Duodenum, Middle Ear, Shoulder, Elbow, CNS, S-I joint, foot, toes	Loneliness, Acute Grief, Humiliated, Trapped, Inhibited, Lack Joy, Greed, Not lovable
2	Pancreas, Stomach	Sinus: Maxillary, Oropharynx, Larynx — Right Breast	Anxiety, Self-Punishment, Broken Power, Hate, Low self-worth, Obsessed
3	Pancreas, Stomach	Sinus: Maxillary, Oropharynx, Larynx — Right Breast	Anxiety, Self-Punishment, Broken Power, Hate, Low self-worth, Obsessed
4	Lung, Large Intestine	Sinus: Paranasal and Ethmoid, Bronchus, Nose	Chronic Grief, Overcritical, Sadness, Controlling, Feeling trapped, Dogmatic, Compulsive, Uptight
5	Lung, Large Intestine	Sinus: Paranasal and Ethmoid, Bronchus, Nose	Chronic Grief, Overcritical, Sadness, Controlling, Feeling trapped, Dogmatic, Compulsive, Uptight
6	Liver, Gallbladder	Sinus: Sphenoid, Palatine Tonsil; Hip, Eye, Knee	Anger, Resentment, Frustration, Blaming, Incapable to take action, Manipulative
7	Kidney, Bladder	Sinus: Frontal, Pharyngeal Tonsil; Genito-Urinary System	Fear, Shame, Guilt, Broken will, Shyness, Helpless, Deep exhaustion
8	Kidney, Bladder	Sinus: Frontal, Pharyngeal Tonsil; Genito-Urinary System	Fear, Shame, Guilt, Broken will, Shyness, Helpless, Deep exhaustion
9	Kidney, Bladder	Sinus: Frontal, Pharyngeal Tonsil; Genito-Urinary System	Fear, Shame, Guilt, Broken will, Shyness, Helpless, Deep exhaustion
10	Kidney, Bladder	Sinus: Frontal, Pharyngeal Tonsil; Genito-Urinary System	Fear, Shame, Guilt, Broken will, Shyness, Helpless, Deep exhaustion
11	Liver, Gallbladder	Sinus: Sphenoid, Palatine Tonsil; Hip, Eye, Knee	Anger, Resentment, Frustration, Blaming, Incapable to take action, Manipulative
12	Lung, Large Intestine	Sinus: Paranasal and Ethmoid, Bronchus, Nose	Chronic Grief, Overcritical, Sadness, Controlling, Feeling trapped, Dogmatic, Compulsive, Uptight
13	Spleen, Stomach	Sinus: Maxillary, Larynx, Lymph, Oropharynx; Knee — Left Breast	Anxiety, Self-Punishment, Broken Power, Hate, Low self-worth, Obsessed
14	Lung, Large Intestine	Sinus: Maxillary, Oropharynx, Larynx — Left Breast	Anxiety, Self-Punishment, Broken Power, Hate, Low self-worth, Obsessed
15	Stomach, Spleen	Sinus: Maxillary, Oropharynx, Larynx — Left Breast	Anxiety, Self-Punishment, Broken Power, Hate, Low self-worth, Obsessed
16	Heart, Small Int., Circulation/Sex, Endocrine	Ileum, Jejunum, Middle Ear, Shoulder, Elbow, CNS, S-I joint, foot, toes	Loneliness, Acute Grief, Humiliated, Trapped, Inhibited, Lack Joy, Greed, Not lovable

Lower Teeth

Tooth #	Organ	Sinus / Body Correlations	Emotions
17	Heart, Small Int., Circulation/Sex, Endocrine	Shoulder, Elbow, Ileum, Jejunum, Peripheral Nerves, S-I joint, foot, toes	Loneliness, Acute Grief, Humiliated, Trapped, Inhibited, Lack Joy, Greed, Not lovable
18	Lung, Large Intestine	Sinus: Paranasal and Ethmoid, Bronchus, Nose	Chronic Grief, Overcritical, Sadness, Controlling, Feeling trapped, Dogmatic, Compulsive, Uptight
19	Large Intestine, Lung	Sinus: Paranasal and Ethmoid, Bronchus, Nose	Chronic Grief, Overcritical, Sadness, Controlling, Feeling trapped, Dogmatic, Compulsive, Uptight
20	Spleen, Stomach	Sinus: Maxillary, Larynx, Lymph, Oropharynx; Knee — Left Breast	Anxiety, Self-Punishment, Broken Power, Hate, Low self-worth, Obsessed
21	Spleen, Stomach	Sinus: Maxillary, Larynx, Lymph, Oropharynx; Knee — Left Breast	Anxiety, Self-Punishment, Broken Power, Hate, Low self-worth, Obsessed
22	Liver, Gallbladder	Sinus: Sphenoid, Palatine Tonsil; Hip, Eye, Knee	Anger, Resentment, Frustration, Blaming, Incapable to take action, Manipulative
23	Kidney, Bladder	Sinus: Frontal, Ear, Pharyngeal Tonsil; Genito-Urinary System	Fear, Shame, Guilt, Broken will, Shyness, Helpless, Deep exhaustion
24	Kidney, Bladder	Sinus: Frontal, Ear, Pharyngeal Tonsil; Genito-Urinary System	Fear, Shame, Guilt, Broken will, Shyness, Helpless, Deep exhaustion
25	Kidney, Bladder	Sinus: Frontal, Ear, Pharyngeal Tonsil; Genito-Urinary System	Fear, Shame, Guilt, Broken will, Shyness, Helpless, Deep exhaustion
26	Kidney, Bladder	Sinus: Frontal, Ear, Pharyngeal Tonsil; Genito-Urinary System	Fear, Shame, Guilt, Broken will, Shyness, Helpless, Deep exhaustion
27	Liver, Gallbladder	Sinus: Sphenoid, Palatine Tonsil; Hip, Eye, Knee	Anger, Resentment, Frustration, Blaming, Incapable to take action, Manipulative
28	Pancreas, Stomach	Sinus: Maxillary, Larynx, Oropharynx; Knee — Right Breast	Anxiety, Self-Punishment, Broken Power, Hate, Low self-worth, Obsessed
29	Pancreas, Stomach	Sinus: Maxillary, Larynx, Oropharynx; Knee — Right Breast	Anxiety, Self-Punishment, Broken Power, Hate, Low self-worth, Obsessed
30	Lung, Large Intestine	Sinus: Paranasal and Ethmoid, Bronchus, Nose	Chronic Grief, Overcritical, Sadness, Controlling, Feeling trapped, Dogmatic, Compulsive, Uptight
31	Lung, Large Intestine	Sinus: Paranasal and Ethmoid, Bronchus, Nose	Chronic Grief, Overcritical, Sadness, Controlling, Feeling trapped, Dogmatic, Compulsive, Uptight
32	Heart, Small Int., Circulation/Sex, Endocrine	Shoulder, Elbow, Ileum, Middle Ear, Peripheral Nerves, S-I joint, foot, toes	Loneliness, Acute Grief, Humiliated, Trapped, Inhibited, Lack Joy, Greed, Not lovable

Abridged, from various sources – credits on website.
Dr. Ralph Wilson   www.NaturalWorldHealing.com

even from the best dentists—some infections don't show up on standard X-rays. You can have a pearly white smile and pink, healthy gums yet still have a massive infection under a crown or in the empty cavity where you had a tooth pulled. I know this all too well from personal experience. The bad news is that unless a dentist is specifically trained to identify these hidden wellness zappers, they are left to fester—creating a lifetime of unnecessary physical and emotional suffering.

As biological dentist extraordinaire Dr. Hal Huggins told me himself as he read from a paper soon to be published, "How many people know the consequences of housing the 40 anaerobic bacteria in implants, the 60 in root canals, or the 8 in cavitations (holes in the jawbones from pulled teeth)? How many know the adverse consequences of trying to fight these microbes with antibiotics? Should you be told the consequences, or just accept the fact that dentistry has raised the requirement bar of 30 million root canals per year up to 60 million per year?" Dr. Huggins firmly believes that root canals are related to serious diseases—MS, leukemia, and breast cancer.

What to do? The good news is that there are dentists trained to look for and treat bacterial infections from the gums and or teeth. I recommend that you check out Dr. Huggins's Web site, where you will find he has an alliance of doctors who are familiar with the safe way to eradicate these problems, so you don't end up sicker than you were beforehand (which is often the case due to the endotoxins that the bacteria produce). (See resources, page 262.)

The next step is to include oil pulling as part of your daily oral hygiene habits. A 2007 study published in the *Journal of Oral Health and Community Dentistry* demonstrated that oil pulling is a very simple yet efficient way to reduce gingivitis by 52 to 60 percent and to reduce plaque by 18 to 30 percent.[2] By the way, oil pulling also beat both mouthwash (which reduces gingivitis by 13 percent and plaque by 20 to 26 percent) and toothbrushing (which reduces gingivitis by 8 to 23 percent and plaque by 11 to 27 percent). And this is just the tip of the iceberg.

Bacteria that are lodged in your mouth can impact virtually every part of your body. That is why it is so crucial to get at the source of these germs so that they do not seep into the rest of your system.

By practicing oil pulling, you get to the root cause of these microscopic invaders and you are involved in germ warfare at the primary site of the invasion. Oil pulling is an Ayurvedic technique that utilizes the dietary oils of Winter Fat Flush (sesame or coconut oil) to pull bacteria, toxins, and mucus out of your mouth. According to Dr. Bruce Fife in his book *Oil Pulling Therapy*, "When you put oil into your mouth, the fatty membranes of the microorganisms are attracted to it. As you swish the oil around your teeth and gums, microbes are picked up as though they are being drawn to a powerful magnet. Bacteria hiding under crevices in the gums and in pores and tubules within the teeth are sucked out of their hiding places and held firmly in the solution. The longer you push and pull the oil through your mouth, the more microbes are pulled free. After twenty minutes, the solution is filled with bacteria, viruses, and other organisms. This is why you want to spit it out rather than swallow it."[3]

This quick and easy morning practice will support the health of your entire body.
Here's what to do:

- Put about 2 teaspoons of oil (such as sesame oil) in your mouth.
- Work the oil around in your mouth for 20 minutes, sloshing it from side to side, sucking and pulling it through your teeth. You can spit out intermittently but make sure you put more oil back in your mouth to continue the process.
- Spit it all out.
- Rinse with a large glass of water to remove any oil residues.

Aromatherapy Baths (20 minutes, 3 times a week before bed)

Hot baths are an excellent way to reduce stress, soothe muscles, care for skin, and encourage detox by opening the pores and stimulating lymph flow—releasing toxins through perspiration. Adding essential oils supercharges your bath by adding the benefits of aromatherapy. Essential oils are distilled from flowers, leaves, and roots of wild or organically grown plants. They quickly absorb into your skin and inhale through your nose, sending a soothing message to the portion of your brain that initiates feelings of well-being and harmony. Benefits include reduced water retention and fat deposits, reduced cortisol levels, reduced muscle soreness, and increased beneficial deep sleep.

It is important to check the label when buying essential oils. The label should state that the oils have been gas chromatograph/mass spectrometer (GC/MS) analyzed to ensure safety and effectiveness. This is really the only way to know that they are high quality and do not include any petrochemicals, fractions of cheaper oils, synthetic fragrance, or other degrading chemicals.

I recommend adding ten drops of an essential oil to a hot bath. Soak for twenty minutes (at the end of the day)—you can combine oils but do not use more than a total of ten drops. During winter, try using oils such as rose and lavender that will help reduce cravings and stress, or rosemary that can help reduce muscular aches, pains, and even arthritis. You may also want to try:

- Sandalwood—promotes inner calm, helping to offset stress and relax the adrenals; encourages deeper sleep
- Thyme—builds immunity
- Geranium—antibacterial, antispasmodic, antitumoral, adrenal support, anti-inflammatory, astringent, antifungal
- Marjoram—calms and helps to reduce stress

You can extend the benefits of essential oils by putting them on cold lightbulbs in lamps in your home or office (when the light is turned on, the heat of the bulb will act as a diffuser of the scent), in oil diffusers, and directly on your skin (such as on your wrists or other pulse points).

10 WINTER FITNESS PLAN

WINTER IS THE SEASON IN WHICH YOU CONSUME the most Clean Carbs, so the workouts are about to become a bit more intense. A major distinguishing feature of the new winter cardio workouts is interval training. Research has shown that interval training yields better and faster weight-loss results than other types of exercise. Interval training allows your body to do more work in a shorter amount of time, by interspersing short bursts of high-intensity exercise with rest or lighter intensity. A study conducted by Laval University in Quebec shows that this method can help you can burn fat five to nine times faster!

Believe it or not, the hardest thing your body does when working out is to warm up and then cool down. During interval training you are constantly using this process; therefore you yield a much greater calorie burn. Think about it for a minute. When you are running, the hardest part is getting started. When you do intervals, you are using muscle glycogen as an energy source, which forces your body to search for fat stores to use. Interval training seems to lessen the risk of muscle loss and may actually increase lean muscle mass, your innate calorie burner.

As you take a look at the workout summary, you'll note that Winter Fitness includes five days of Yoga-Quickies and Cardio Workouts plus three nonconsecutive days of core training. Make sure you give your muscles a recovery day during the Core Exercises. Ironically, it is during this rest period that your muscle actually tones so that when you do work out, you are benefiting the most from your exercise routine. Whatever you do, do not overexercise (two or more hours a day). Exercise places good stress on the body, but when done in excess, it causes your cortisol levels to rise, overstimulates the adrenals, and can actually decrease the amount of fat you burn. The bottom line is: don't "excessercise."

> *My back and knee pain from past injuries have disappeared and my energy levels have soared. I can now work out several times a week and don't get winded on long hikes like some of my hunting buddies.*
>
> —*Tim, Fat Flush Fan*

Although it may be cold outside, don't be afraid to embrace other physical activities that allow you to enjoy some fresh air from time to time. For instance, you can offset the falling temperatures outside by keeping your core temperature heated up with outdoor winter cardio such as skiing, snowshoeing, or shoveling snow.

Winter Workout Summary

Yoga-Quickies *(5 to 10 minutes, 5 days a week; turn to page 49 in the Pre–Fat Flush Fitness Plan for a description of these moves.)*
Yoga-Quickie Belly Breathing
Yoga-Quickie Calming Breath
Yoga-Quickie Poses (1 to 5)

Winter Cardio Workouts *(45 minutes for Workouts 1 and 2; 25 minutes for Workout 3; 5 days a week, select Workout 1, 2, or 3)*
Workout 1—Walkout for the Treadmill
Workout 2—A Walk in the Park Cardio Interval Training
Workout 3—Rebounding

Winter Core Exercises *(5 to 10 minutes, 3 nonconsecutive days a week)*
Medicine Ball Crunch
Torso Twist
Side Plank
Back Extension

WINTER CARDIO WORKOUTS

With the exception of rebounding, you'll need to set aside 45 minutes (including warm-ups and cool-downs) for these workouts. Keep in mind that the specified 25 minutes of rebounding is roughly equivalent to 45 minutes of the other two cardio options. Follow the Rate of Perceived Exertion (RPE) Scale (see page 57).

Cardio Option 1—Walkout for the Treadmill

Duration: 45 minutes
Frequency: 5 days a week
Targets: Cardiovascular and lymphatic systems
Body-Shaping Tools: Walking shoes

Cardio Option 2—A Walk in the Park Interval Training

Duration: 45 minutes; follow instructions for each segment as indicated
Frequency: 5 days a week
Targets: Cardiovascular and lymphatic systems and full body toning
Body-Shaping Tools: Walking shoes

This routine combines cardio interval training with toning. You can do this workout either outdoors or, if it's too cold, on the treadmill.

Walkout for the Treadmill Routine

Warm-Up Walk	5 minutes; RPE 3–4
Walk	3 minutes, increase speed to 3.5 mph; RPE 5–6
Sprint or Walk or Run	1 minute; RPE 8–9
Walk	5 minutes, decrease speed to 2.8 mph; increase incline to 8 (pump your arms as you climb); RPE 7–8
Walk	3 minutes, increase speed to 3.8 mph; decrease incline to 0; RPE 6–7
Sprint or Walk or Run	1 minute; RPE 8–9
Walk	5 minutes; decrease speed to 3 mph; increase incline to 5 (pump your arms as you climb); RPE 7–8
Walk	5 minutes; increase speed to 3.5 mph; decrease incline to 0; RPE 3–4
Sprint or Walk or Run	1 minute; RPE 8–9
Walk	5 minutes; decrease speed to 2.6 mph; increase incline to 10 (pump your arms as you climb); RPE 8–9
Walk	5 minutes; increase speed to 3.8 mph; decrease incline to 0; RPE 6–7
Sprint or Walk or Run	1 minute; RPE 8–9
Cool-Down Walk	5 minutes; RPE 3–4

Total Workout Time: 45 minutes, including warm-up and cool-down.

Warm-Up Segment—Walking
Duration: 5 minutes; RPE 1–3

Cardio Toning Segment 1—Alternating Lunges
Duration: 1 minute; RPE 5–6

Stand with your feet together. Take a large step (approximately 2 to 3 feet) forward with your right foot. Bend your knees and lower your upper body while keeping your torso upright, shoulders back, and abdominals in for strength. Keep your knee behind your toes as you come down, then return to the starting position by driving through the heel of your lead foot (right foot). Step the left foot next to the right and then repeat the movements with your left foot.

Cardio Segment 1—Walking
Duration: 5 minutes; RPE 3–4

Cardio Toning Segment 2—Park Push-ups
Duration: 1 minute; 12 to 15 repetitions; RPE 5–6

Start by standing a few feet away from a tree. Lean forward at a diagonal, with your arms out straight, and place your hands shoulder-width apart on the tree. Bring your chest in toward the tree by bending your elbows, then press back to starting position. Make sure to maintain a straight line with your body.

Cardio Segment 2—Walking
Duration: 5 minutes; RPE 4–5

Cardio Toning Segment 3—Side Lunges
Duration: 1 minute; 12 to 15 repetitions; RPE 5–6
    Stand with your feet together. Keeping your left leg straight, take a wide step out to the side with your right leg. Lean slightly forward from the hips as you bend your right knee into a lunge position (keeping your right knee over your ankle and behind your toes). Push off the right leg to return to the starting position. Repeat with opposite side.

Cardio Segment 3—Speed Walk or Run
Duration: 5 minutes; RPE 6–7
Speed walk or run at a brisk pace, pumping your arms. If possible, walk or run up and down hills.

Cardio Toning Segment 4—Park Bench Dips
Duration: 1 minute; 12–15 repetitions; RPE 5–6
Body-Shaping Tools: Bench
    Start by sitting on the edge of a bench. Place your hands palm down and shoulder-width apart on the edge of the bench. Walk your feet out to a bent knee position while keeping a straight back and shoulders in line with your hips. Lower your body into a dip by bending your elbows and then press back up to starting position. To prevent placing excessive stress on the shoulders, be sure not to let your shoulders dip down any lower than elbow height.

Cardio Segment 4—Speed Walk or Run
Duration: 5 minutes; RPE 6–7
    Speed walk or run at a brisk pace, pumping your arms. Try to find hills to walk up and down.

Cardio Toning Segment 5—Skipping
Duration: 1 minute; RPE 5–6
    Be sure to pump your arms and legs vigorously while skipping, to get the lymph flowing.

Cardio Segment 6—Walking
Duration: 5 minutes; RPE 3–4

Cardio Toning Segment 6—Skipping
Duration: 1 minute; RPE 5–6

Cardio Toning Segment 7—Mountain Climbers
Duration: 1 minute; RPE 7–8
Place your hands shoulder-width apart on a bench or the ground. Step both feet back into a basic push-up position. Bring one foot forward toward your chest while keeping the other leg straight back. Place your weight on the balls of your feet. Briskly shift the legs back and forth as if you are climbing.

Cardio Segment 7—Speed Walk or Run
Duration: 7 minutes; RPE 7–8
Speed walk or run, pumping your arms. Incorporate hills if possible.

Cardio Toning Segment 8—Alternating Knee Lifts
Duration: 1 minute; RPE 5–6
Stand with your feet together. Place your hands on your shoulders with your elbows out. Raise your right knee toward your left elbow. Bring your leg back down. Repeat movement with the opposite leg and knee.

Cool-Down Segment
Duration: 5 minutes; RPE 1–3
Walk at a slower pace to bring your heart rate to the cool-down stretch levels.

Total Workout Time: 45 minutes, including warm-up and cool-down

Cardio Option 3—Rebounding
Duration: 25 minutes, including warm-up and cool-down (to the beat of your favorite iPod tunes)
Frequency: Five days a week
Targets: Cardiovascular and lymphatic systems
Body-Shaping Tools: Rebounder

Twist Bounce with Blade Arms
With your feet together or apart, twist your torso in the opposite direction of your lower body while moving your arms overhead in a scissorlike motion.

Front Kicks with Alternating Arms

With your feet together, bounce and kick one foot forward, alternating arms forward.

Heel-Jack Bounce with Alternating Arms

Start with your feet together and then bounce by taking only one heel out at a time and, simultaneously on the same side, circling one arm back.

Rebounding Routine

Warm-Up Light Bounce—5 minutes
Cardio Phase—15 minutes
   Front Kicks with Alternating Arms—4 minutes
   Heel-Jack Bounce with Alternating Arms—4 minutes
   Twist Bounce with Blade Arms—4minutes
   Jumping Jack Bounce—3 minutes
Cool-Down Light Bounce—5 minutes
Total Workout Time: 25 minutes, including warm-up and cool-down

CORE EXERCISES

When talking about the core most people automatically think of just their abs. Your core actually encompasses a much larger area than you think. The muscles of the core run the entire length of the trunk and torso—twenty-nine muscles, to be exact. You could pretty much draw a line all the way around the body from the top of your rib cage to about midthigh. This area has often been referred to as your "powerhouse." Weak and unbalanced core muscles are often a leading cause of lower back pain. A strong stable core will make almost all of your physical activities easier.

The following exercises will strengthen your core. It is typical to feel your lower back engaged during core work. The ultimate goal is to strengthen the lower back, so you will definitely want to start with just a few seconds of each exercise and build up gradually. As you increase strength you will be able to hold the positions longer.

The upcoming exercises utilize a medicine ball, stability ball, or BOSU Balance Trainer (see resources, page 259). Generally speaking, the stability ball and BOSU are going to add more of an element of balance and core stabilization, making exercises slightly more difficult to fire up fat burning. The medicine ball is a weighted ball that comes in many different weights and sizes. I recommend a 6-pound medicine ball for women and a 10-pound ball for men.

Core Training Tips
1. Remember to focus on the quality of your movements instead of on the amount of repetitions you do. Each movement should be slow and controlled.
2. Don't hold your breath; continue breathing steadily throughout.
3. Make sure to allow a day between core training workouts, as the core muscles are no different than any other muscles and they need time to recover.

Medicine Ball Crunch
Duration: 1 set of 10
Frequency: 3 nonconsecutive days per week
Targets: Rectus abdominals
Body-Shaping Tools: Medicine ball (6-pound ball for women, 10-pound ball for men); BOSU (optional)

    Lie on your back on a mat or a BOSU, and hold a medicine ball with your arms fully extended overhead. Keep your arms close to your head while doing an

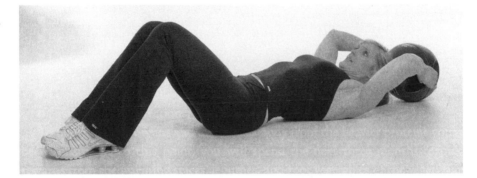

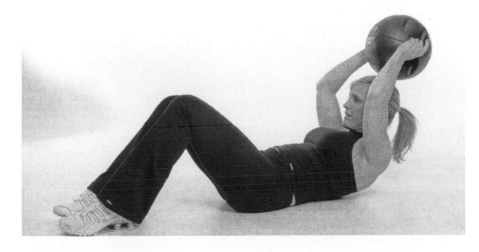

abdominal crunch. As you come up, keep your chin slightly tucked in. Don't let the ball move past your head; keep it stationary and overhead.

Torso Twist

Duration: 1 set of 10; do set 3 times
Frequency: 3 nonconsecutive days per week
Targets: Core
Body-Shaping Tools: Stability ball and medicine ball

Sit securely on the stability ball. Hold the medicine ball at your side. Twist the ball diagonally across your body with straight arms to an overhead position on the opposite side of your body. Then in the same manner, twist downward to bring the ball back to the starting position.

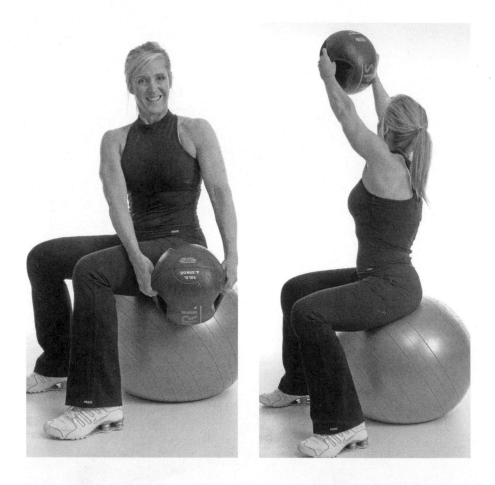

Side Plank

Duration: 1 set of 10; do set 3 times

Frequency: 3 nonconsecutive days per week

Targets: Transverse abdominals, obliques, abductors, core

Body-Shaping Tool: BOSU

Lie on the BOSU on your side; place your elbow in the middle of the BOSU directly under your shoulder. Put one foot in front of the other. Engage your core and press into position, remembering to squeeze your glutes and keep your body in a straight line.

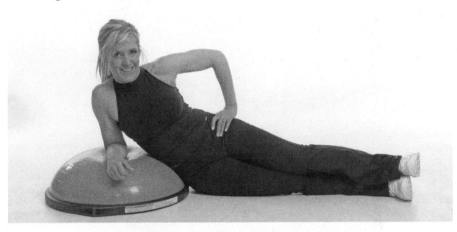

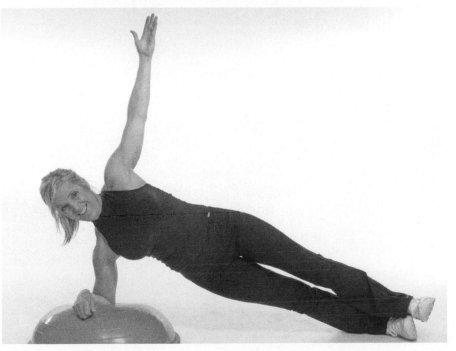

Back Extension

Duration: 1 set of 10; do set 3 times

Frequency: 3 days per week total

Targets: Lower back, erector spinae, and glutes

Body-Shaping Tool: Stability ball

Lie on the stability ball on your abdomen, a little past the middle of the ball, with your feet hip-distance apart. Place your hands behind your head, engage your glutes, lower your back, and lift your torso—try not to hyperextend.

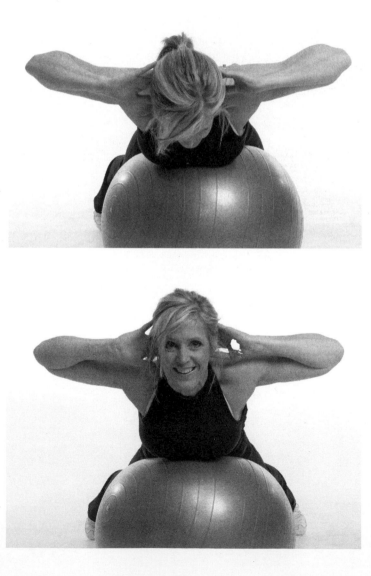

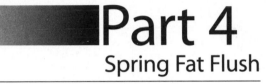

Part 4
Spring Fat Flush

11 SPRING FAT FLUSH DIET

*Persistence and determination alone are omnipotent. The slogan
"press on" has solved and always will solve the problems of the
human race.*

—Calvin Coolidge

BY NOW, YOU WILL HAVE ACHIEVED some impressive results. You've
already lost a good deal of weight and inches. You got rid of unwanted tummy fat.
You are more flexible and limber than you have been in years. And you've finally
started to see some changes for the better in your cellulite. You are ready to shift
gears into Spring Fat Flush.

In spring, the world is reawakening and coming into bloom with renewed
energy. Nutrient-rich greens are the hallmark of the season. This is the best time
of the year to turn attention to your liver and its sister organ, the gallbladder.
Your liver, after all, is your body's major detoxifier and key to life. When your
liver is sluggish, more than four hundred bodily processes are affected. Seasonal
symptoms that relate to the liver and gallbladder include:

- Rib cage sensitivity, particularly under the right ribs
- Chronic tension in the neck and across the shoulders
- Feeling tired and sleepy after eating
- Waking up between 1:00 and 3:00 a.m.
- Nausea, especially after eating fatty foods
- Light-colored stools
- Hormonal imbalances from perimenopause to menopause with hot flashes
- PMS irritability, bloating

To safely nourish and support this vital organ, the Spring Fat Flush diet eliminates dairy and some of the heavier winter foods from your meal plan. It focuses
on cleansing foods that allow the liver to function more effectively to emulsify fat
and keep you slim and trim yearlong. In other words, it's time to take your detox
to the next level.

In Spring Fat Flush you will continue with the Cranberry H_2O, which contains powerful phytochemicals and organic acids that stimulate the release of
trapped fats, fluids, and toxins. You will also continue to consume the daily Green
Life Cocktail as you still can benefit from this green superfood mixture, rich in
detoxifying nutrients.

You'll find many of the delicious Fat Flushing Superstar foods from Winter Fat Flush are still on the menu, including Clean Carb choices such as sweet potatoes, green peas, carrots, winter squash, Ezekiel 4:9 tortillas, and French Meadow Healthseed Spelt Bread. However, you will also find that some foods have lost their "Superstar" status, such as legumes and crackers, as well as nuts and seeds, because we are progressing into a more stringent detox eating program that will also supercharge weight loss. Dairy, with the exception of whey protein—which most individuals can tolerate if it is undenatured and unheated; it does not contain the allergens casein and lactose of regular milk products—is also off the list because it increases mucus production, which you want to avoid in the spring. In essence, you are counteracting the moisture of spring with a choice of drier foods.

The pounds may start to pare off even more rapidly due to your lighter diet and your continued workout program. The duration of your fitness routines will lessen slightly, but you will still be strength-training and building muscle mass, the body's most metabolically active tissue, so you will be burning more calories, even while you are resting. Although results do vary, you can expect to lose one or two pounds and another two to three inches per week.

Unfortunately, the less you need to lose, the slower the weight comes off. If you feel your weight loss is stalled, about three weeks into Spring Fat Flush you may want to incorporate the 5-Day Hot Metabolism Booster Plan (see page 251).

To make weight-loss go even more smoothly, I am providing you with two weeks of sample meal plans to help get you started.

Oh, and one more thing: Watch your brew. Both beer and wine are no-no's because they are notoriously yeast-provoking. Beer drinkers have the highest waist-to-hip ratios of those who have six or more drinks a week, according to University

Teas and Herbs that Cleanse, Heal, and Relax

Dandelion root tea is the premier springtime herbal tea. It provides gentle liver decongesting by stimulating bile and helps to alleviate liver inflammation. If the liver or gallbladder symptoms resonate with you, drink one to two cups a day.

Liver-protecting herbs include gentian root, which stimulates the gallbladder to increase secretion and flush out bacteria; milk thistle, an antioxidant-rich herb that protects and helps rejuvenate the liver; yellow dock, a time-honored liver purifier and toner; and Oregon grape root, helpful in clearing up secondary skin conditions such as acne and psoriasis, which are connected to a toxic liver. Several of these herbs are included in the Weight Loss Formula supplement that is part of the Fat Flush Kit.

of North Carolina research. Remember this motto: overgrowth = overweight. (Sorry—I have a dark field microscope in my office and have viewed too many blood samples from wine and beer drinkers not to notice the overabundance of yeast buds.) Not so with potato vodka, tequila, and rum (made from sugar), so a shot glass on weekends or for special events while you are on Spring Fat Flush is A-okay as long as you don't go overboard.

> *I've lost 19.5 pounds since I started on December 7. I've lost a total of 14.25 inches. It is truly amazing what takes place during this process. Even though I started…at a very busy time, it was perfect for me to start in December and get through the holidays. Now, it is only getting better.*
>
> *—Fat Flush online fan*

SPRING FAT FLUSHING SUPERSTAR FOODS

Here you will find healthy eating choices that will make menu planning for Spring Fat Flush more personalized. Clean Carbs will continue to provide a treasure chest of phytonutrients such as carotenoids (sweet potatoes), fiber (bread and tortillas), and cancer-fighting isothiocyanates (rutabagas and turnips) that will enable you to eat better and feel better while losing weight. However, since you're stepping up your detox, some Winter Fat Flushing Superstar Foods are no longer on the list. On the bright side, I've added some alcohol—in moderation, of course—to lift your spirits.

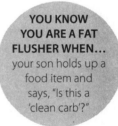

YOU KNOW YOU ARE A FAT FLUSHER WHEN… your son holds up a food item and says, "Is this a 'clean carb'?"

Cranberry H$_2$O
Recipe: See page 198.
Bodily Consumption: 64 ounces per day between each meal and snack, in Green Life Cocktail, and in frappés.

Spiced Lemon Toddy
Recipe: See page 200.
Bodily Consumption: daily on arising

Green Life Cocktail
Recipe: See page 199.
Bodily Consumption: Daily on arising

Probiotic Sweetener
Benefits: Contains beneficial bacteria to balance GI tract for weight-loss insurance and enhanced immunity. Provides yeast-free sweetener for no-heat frappés, beverages, and desserts.
Brand: UNI KEY's Flora-Key
Bodily Consumption: 2 to 3 teaspoons per day in Green Life Cocktails, frappés, and with nonheated foods

Whey Protein
Benefits: Assists lean muscle mass development, increases energy, natural appetite suppressant
Brands: UNI KEY's Fat Flush Vanilla or Chocolate Whey Protein
Bodily Consumption: Up to 2 servings per day (20 grams protein each) in frappés, muffins, desserts, whey pancakes, etc. Note: Chocolate whey is limited to 2 servings per week.

Chia Seeds
Bodily Consumption: 2 to 3 tablespoons per day, added to frappés, soups, stews, and dressings or sprinkled on such foods as eggs and veggies

Slimming Oils
Choose from:
High-lignan Flaxseed Oil
Bodily Consumption: Total of 2 tablespoons per day of flaxseed oil and/or fish oil. Do not heat flaxseed oil.

Fish Oil
Bodily Consumption: Total of 2 tablespoons per day of flaxseed oil and/or fish oil. Do not heat fish oil.

Extra-Virgin Olive Oil in an oil mister (such as Misto).
Bodily Consumption: Lightly spritz in cooking as needed.

Herbs, Spices, and Seasonings
Choose from:

Anise
Apple cider vinegar
Basil (fresh or dried)
Bay leaves (fresh or dried)
Cayenne
Chinese five-spice powder
Chives (fresh or dried)
Cilantro
Cloves
Coriander
Cream of tartar
Cumin
Dijon mustard (without added sugar)
Dill (fresh or dried)

Dry mustard
Fennel (fresh or dried)
Garlic (fresh or garlic powder)
Ginger (fresh or dried)
Mint (fresh or dried)
Onion powder
Oregano (fresh or dried)
Parsley (fresh or dried)
Rosemary (fresh or dried)
Turmeric
Wasabi

Bodily Consumption: ¼ to ½ teaspoon at least 3 to 5 times per week

Protein
Bodily Consumption: a minimum of 8 ounces of cooked lean protein
Choose from:
Suggested varieties of canned and fresh fish, shellfish and seafood (wild encouraged)
Lean beef, lamb, veal (organic/grass-fed encouraged), and other meats
Poultry
Omega-enriched eggs (hormone-free/free-range encouraged)
Vegetarian Protein Sources: Tofu and tempeh

Fish
Choose from:
Fresh

Bass
Cod
Grouper
Haddock
Halibut
Mackerel
Mahimahi
Orange roughy
Perch
Pike
Pollock
Salmon
Sardines
Snapper
Sole
Squid
Trout

Tuna
Whitefish
Canned
Crabmeat
(Featherweight,
Seasons, Lillie, Three
Star)
Light tuna—not
albacore (Natural
Sea, Crown Prince)

Mackerel   Olhao, Crown   Crab
Salmon (Natural   Prince)   Lobster
Sea, Crown Prince,   Scallops
Vital Choice)   *Shellfish*   Shrimp
Sardines (Bela,   Calamari

Meat
Choose from:
Lean beef, lamb, veal, and other meats

Beef   *Lamb*   *Other Meats*
  Brisket   Leg   Elk
  Chuck   Loin   Ostrich
  Eye of round   Rib   Venison
  Flank   Bison from Hole
  London broil   *Veal*   Buffalo Company
  Round   Loin   (www.jhbuffalomeat
  Rump   Rib   .com) and Buffalo
                      Shoulder   Gal (www.buffalogal
                                        .com)

Poultry
Choose from:
White meat of skinned turkey and chicken, fresh or frozen. Look for free-range and hormone-free, such as Foster Farms, Harmony Farms, Shelton Farms, and Young Farms.

In addition to the above protein choices you may also enjoy:

Omega-Enriched Eggs
Bodily Consumption: Up to 2 per day

Vegetarian Protein Sources
Choose from:
   Tofu—unflavored, firm and silken (Mori-Nu, White Wave)
   Tempeh (Turtle Island Foods, Lightlife)
Bodily Consumption: Up to 2 servings (4 ounces each) of tofu and/or tempeh
   per week

Fruits

Benefits: These low-glycemic fruits are high in vitamin C, natural enzymes, muscle-sparing potassium, and are the best natural snacks on the planet. Look for fresh (without mold) or frozen.

Brands (frozen): Cascadian Farm (www.cfarm.com) or Stahlbush Farms (www.stahlbush.com)

Bodily Consumption: Up to 2 servings per day

Choose from:

1 small apple, orange, nectarine, peach, pear, or pomegranate	6 large strawberries
1 cup berries (blueberries, blackberries, raspberries, and/or cranberries)	10 large cherries
	2 medium-size plums
	½ grapefruit
	Lemons and limes (as desired)

Vegetables

Fresh: Look for fresh (in season locally is best) vegetables that are full of vibrant color so that you can eat the rainbow.

Brands (canned): No added salt or sugar

Brands (frozen): Frozen vegetables are acceptable as well, such as Woodstock Farms (www.woodstock-farms.com), Cascadian Farm (www.cfarm.com), and Stahlbush Farm (www.stahlbush.com).

Bodily Consumption: Aim for at least 5 or more servings per day.

A vegetable serving is generally 1 cup raw or ½ cup cooked.

Choose from:

(*All unlimited except where noted*)	Carrots (limit 1 medium-size or 5 baby)	Endive
Artichokes (1 whole or 5 hearts)	Cauliflower	Escarole
Arugula	Celery	Green beans
Asparagus	Celery root	Hearts of palm
Bamboo shoots	Chard	Jalapeños
Bell peppers (red, green, and orange)	Chinese cabbage	Jerusalem artichoke
Bok choy	Chives	Jicama
Broccoli	Cilantro	Kale
Brussels sprouts	Collard greens	Kohlrabi
Burdock	Cucumbers	Leeks
Cabbage	Daikon	Lettuce (red or green, romaine, butter, baby greens, etc.)
	Dandelion greens	Mushrooms
	Eggplant	

Mustard greens	Sprouts (alfalfa,	*Tomato Products (no*
Okra	mung bean, broccoli)	*added sugar or salt)*
Olives (black, 3 per	Sugar snap peas	Diced tomatoes
day)	Tomatillos	Pizza sauce
Onions	Tomatoes and	Tomato paste
Parsley	tomato products (see	Tomato puree
Radicchio	below)	Tomato sauce
Radishes	Water chestnuts	Whole peeled
Rhubarb (1 cup)	Watercress	tomatoes
Shallots	Yellow squash	*Brands:* Muir Glen,
Snow peas	Zucchini	Eden, Bio Nature,
Spaghetti squash		Woodstock Farms
Spinach		

Sea Vegetables

Benefits: Rich in iodine and many trace minerals such as calcium and iron, sea veggies support thyroid function and also inhibit the absorption of radiation and heavy metals.

Choose from: Agar, arame, hijiki, kombu, nori, sea palm fronds, wakame

Brand: Eden

Bodily Consumption: Up to 2 servings of 1 tablespoon agar and/or ½ cup of arame, hijiki, kombu, nori, sea palm fronds, and wakame per week added to soups, stews, poultry, beef, fish, seafood, salads, veggies, eggs, etc.

You may also add a sea veggie–based seasoning:

Brand: Eden Seaweed Gomasio (contains sea vegetables, sesame seeds, and sea salt)

Bodily Consumption: ½ teaspoon daily

CLEAN CARBS

In the first month, cut back to simply one serving each day of a Clean Carb from either the starchy vegetables or the bread and tortilla groups, to start lightening up your diet. During the second month, add a half serving of another Clean Carb. In the third month, enjoy two servings (total) of a combination of starchy vegetables, bread and tortillas, and selected grains.

Starchy Vegetables (cooked)

Choose from:

1 small sweet potato or yam	½ cup winter squash (such as
½ cup green peas	butternut, Delicata, hubbard,
½ cup carrots	acorn, and kabocha)
	½ cup parsnips

½ cup turnips

½ cup rutabagas

½ cup pumpkin (fresh or unsweetened canned)

Bread and Tortillas

Brands: French Meadow Healthseed Spelt Bread (yeast-free), Kinnikinnick Candadi Multi-Grain Rice Bread (yeast- and gluten-free), Food for Life Ezekiel 4:9 Sprouted Grain Tortilla (yeast- and gluten-free)

Bodily Consumption: 1 slice bread or 1 (6-inch) tortilla

Grains and Cereals

Quinoa

Bodily Consumption: ½ cup cooked

Oatmeal (rolled or steel-cut)

Bodily Consumption: ½ cup cooked

Beverages

Healing Tea

Dandelion root

Brands: Alvita, Traditional Medicinals

Bodily Consumption: 1 to 2 cups per day

Legal Cheats

Organic coffee (caffeinated)

Benefits: Provides antioxidants and B vitamins such as niacin

Brands: Newman's Own Organics, Organic Coffee Co.

Bodily Consumption: 1 cup each day

Turkey Bacon

Brand: Applegate Farms

Bodily Consumption: 1 to 2 slices

Alcohol *(grain-free)*

Benefit: Mood lifter

Choose from:

Potato vodka

Rum (made from sugar)

Tequila (from the cactus plant)

Bodily Consumption: 1 ounce mixed with water, Cranberry H_2O, or unflavored sparkling water once a week

Sparkling water (unflavored)

Brands: Perrier, San Pellegrino

Bodily Consumption: 8 ounces, 2 to 3 times per week

Salt

Benefits: Aids digestion and acid/
alkaline balance

Brands: Morton's Canning and
Pickling Salt, Real Salt, Himalayan
Pink Salt

Bodily Consumption: ½ to 1 teaspoon
per day. (Use your best judgment—
if you bloat, are hypertensive, or
take a diuretic then take less. If you
have low blood sugar or suffer from
adrenal exhaustion, you can use up
to 1 teaspoon per day.)

Stevia Plus (for use in heated foods)

Bodily Consumption: Maximum of 2
(0.035-ounce or 1-gram) packets
per day

A GENTLE REMINDER—ESPECIALLY FOR SPRING FAT FLUSH

- Menu plans are completely optional. If following a structured plan is not for you, feel free to create your own fabulous Fat Flush–friendly meals and snacks that follow the Spring Fat Flush guidelines.
- Recipes noted with an asterisk (*) appear in chapter 21.
- Lunches, dinners, and snacks are interchangeable within the same day.
- You may add an extra tablespoon of chia seeds into recipes, if desired.
- Continue to drink one Green Life Cocktail daily. You will continue to drink 64 ounces of Cranberry H_2O, unheated now. In addition, you may also enjoy 1 daily cup each of regular coffee and 1 to 2 cups of dandelion root tea.
- Continue to optimize your results with the Fat Flush Kit supplements: the Dieters' Multi (with or without iron) for balanced vitamin and mineral supplementation; the GLA 90s for stimulating brown adipose tissue metabolism, which increases fat burning and keeps skin moist and taut during weight loss; and the Weight Loss Formula for carbohydrate control, fat metabolism, and liver support (without stimulants). Also continue to take 1,000 mg of CLA three times per day with meals.

SPRING FAT FLUSH: 7-DAY SPRING MEAL PLANNER (MONTH 1)

DAY 1

On Arising
Spiced Lemon Toddy* (page 200)
Green Life Cocktail* (page 199)

Breakfast
Pears 'n' Cinnamon Frappé* (page 202)

Snack
2 hard-boiled eggs with a pinch of Seaweed Gomasio

Lunch
Tuna Nori Roll made with 4 ounces of
canned tuna, celery, red pepper, and 2
tablespoons E-Z Classic Mayo* (page
235) rolled in a sheet of nori

*Fat Flush on the Fly: No time to make
homemade mayo? Try 1 tablespoon of
Spectrum's Omega-3 Organic Mayonnaise with Flax Oil.*

Snack
1 apple, sliced and sprinkled with 1 tablespoon of chia seeds

Dinner
4 ounces grilled salmon with lime and Fat
Flush Seasoning* (page 235)
½ cup steamed garden peas with mint
Wilted baby spinach salad with red onion
rings and 1 tablespoon of apple cider
vinegar

*Timesaver Tip! Grill an extra 4 ounces of
salmon for Day 2's Lunch.*

DAY 2

On Arising
Spiced Lemon Toddy* (page 200)
Green Life Cocktail* (page 199)

Breakfast
Two-Egg Scrambler made with red, green,
and orange peppers, with a pinch of
Seaweed Gomasio and 1 tablespoon of
chia seeds
1 orange

Snack
A bowl of chicken broth with diced veggies and a pinch of cayenne

Lunch
Dragon Bowl Salad* (page 219) topped
with 4 ounces of leftover grilled salmon
and 1 tablespoon each of lemon juice
and flaxseed oil

Snack
Blackberry Mojito Tease Frappé* (page 202)

Dinner
4 ounces grilled chicken burger with red
onion and tomato slices, lettuce, and
Dijon mustard
Sautéed mushrooms and water chestnuts
with parsley
½ cup Baked Parsnip Fries* (page 228)

*Fat Flush on the Fly: Murray's Chicken
Express Ground Chicken Burgers*

DAY 3

On Arising
Spiced Lemon Toddy* (page 200)
Green Life Cocktail* (page 199)

Breakfast
2 poached eggs over warm baby spinach
with basil, oregano, and 1 tablespoon
of chia seeds
½ grapefruit with 1 teaspoon Flora-Key

Snack
Jicama sticks with freshly squeezed lime
juice

Lunch
Chef's Salad made with 4 ounces of roasted turkey, mixed greens, cucumber,
tomato, pepper rings, and 2 tablespoons of Herbal Dijon Vinaigrette*
(page 238)

Fat Flush on the Fly: Applegate Farms Roasted Turkey

Snack
Pumpkin Pie Frappé* (page 202)

Dinner
4 ounces broiled shrimp with Fat Flush
Seasoning* (page 235)
Fennel braised in veggie broth and freshly
squeezed lemon juice

Timesaver Tip! Broil an extra 4 ounces shrimp
for Day 4's Lunch.

DAY 4

On Arising
Spiced Lemon Toddy* (page 200)
Green Life Cocktail* (page 199)

Breakfast
Orange Creamsicle Frappé* (page 202)
1 slice Kinnikinnick Rice Bread, toasted

Snack
2 hard-boiled eggs smashed with Dijon
mustard and cilantro

Lunch
Radicchio and endive salad with jicama,
parsley, 4 ounces of leftover grilled
shrimp, and 1 tablespoon each of flaxseed oil and apple cider vinegar

Snack
6 large strawberries with 1 teaspoon
Flora-Key

Dinner
2 cups Szechuan Tofu and Eggplant* (page
221) on a bed of steamed spaghetti
squash and shredded zucchini, with 1
tablespoon of chia seeds

Timesaver Tip! Save leftover tofu with eggplant for Day 5's Lunch.

DAY 5

On Arising
Spiced Lemon Toddy* (page 200)
Green Life Cocktail* (page 199)

Breakfast
2-egg omelet with cremini mushrooms,
green onions, and 1 tablespoon of chia
seeds
1 cup blueberries

Snack
Hearts of palm and 3 artichoke hearts with
dill and freshly squeezed lime juice

Lunch
2 cups leftover Szechuan Tofu with Eggplant* on a bed of warm asparagus

Snack
Just Cherries Frappé* (page 201)

Dinner
4 ounces grilled lamb chops with Fat Flush
Seasoning* (page 235)
½ cup oven-roasted turnips with oregano
Red leaf lettuce salad with grated carrot
and 1 tablespoon each of apple cider
vinegar and flaxseed oil

DAY 6

On Arising
Spiced Lemon Toddy* (page 200)
Green Life Cocktail* (page 199)

Breakfast
Mediterranean Scramble* (page 207)
1 pear, sliced, with ground cinnamon and 1
tablespoon of chia seeds

Snack
A bowl of veggie broth with green onions,
nori strips, and a pinch of cayenne

Lunch
Turkey Burger LettuceWrap made with 4
ounces of grilled turkey burger, Dijon
mustard, red onion, and tomato,
wrapped in a large lettuce leaf

½ cup baked butternut squash with
ground cloves and ginger

*Fat Flush on the Fly: Applegate Farm's
Organic Turkey*

Snack
Tootsie Roll Twist Frappé* (page 202)

Dinner
2 cups Chicken Cacciatore* (page 210)
Oven-roasted Jerusalem artichoke and
leeks with cilantro and 1 tablespoon of
flaxseed oil

*Timesaver Tip! Save leftover Chicken Caccia-
tore for Day 7's Lunch.*

DAY 7

On Arising
Spiced Lemon Toddy* (page 200)
Green Life Cocktail* (page 199)

Breakfast
Peach Melba Frappé* (page 202)
1 Ezekiel 4:9 tortilla, toasted

Snack
¼ cup Lemony Tapenade* (page 248)
Asparagus and endive dippers

Lunch
2 cups leftover Chicken Cacciatore*
Watercress and parsley salad with 2 table-
    spoons of Herbal Dijon Vinaigrette*
    (page 238)

Snack
2 hard-boiled eggs
1 apple

Dinner
4 ounces grilled London broil with Fat
    Flush Seasoning* (page 235)
Steamed kale with lemon zest and 1 table-
    spoon of chia seeds

SPRING FAT FLUSH: 7-DAY SPRING MEAL PLANNER (MONTH 3)

DAY 1

On Arising
Spiced Lemon Toddy* (page 200)
Green Life Cocktail* (page 199)

Breakfast
Blueberry "Cheesecake" Frappé* (page 202)

Snack
2 hard-boiled eggs with a pinch of Sea-
    weed Gomasio

Lunch
On-the-Go Shrimp Lettuce Wraps made
    with 4 ounces of cooked shrimp,
    chopped celery, red onion, and 2 table-
    spoons of Fresh Herbed Mayonnaise*
    (page 235), wrapped in large lettuce
    leaves

*Fat Flush on the Fly: No time to make
    homemade mayo? Try 1 tablespoon of
    Spectrum Omega-3 Mayonnaise with
    Flax Oil.*

Snack
1 Fabulous Chia Crax* (page 246)
1 pear

Dinner
4 ounces Cinnamon-Scented Cranberry
    Brisket* (page 214)
½ cup steamed garden peas with mint and
    baby spinach salad with grated daikon
    radish, cilantro, and 1 tablespoon of
    apple cider vinegar

*Timesaver Tip! Save leftover brisket for Day
    2's Lunch.*

DAY 2

On Arising
Spiced Lemon Toddy* (page 200)
Green Life Cocktail* (page 199)

Breakfast
2 eggs scrambled with red pepper, green
onions, and oregano
1 slice French Meadow Healthseed Spelt
Bread, toasted

Snack
6 large sliced strawberries sprinkled with 1
teaspoon Flora-Key
1 Fabulous Chia Crax* (page 246)

Lunch
4 ounces leftover Cinnamon-Scented Cranberry Brisket*
Mixed baby greens with pea pods, broccoli sprouts, and 1 tablespoon each of
apple cider vinegar and flaxseed oil

Snack
Peaches 'n' Cream Frappé* (page 202)

Dinner
4 ounces grilled mahimahi with freshly
squeezed lemon juice and rosemary
½ cup steamed carrots with a pinch of Seaweed Gomasio
Braised Fragrant Chard* (page 227)

DAY 3

On Arising
Spiced Lemon Toddy* (page 200)
Green Life Cocktail* (page 199)

Breakfast
Egg, Portobello, and Spinach Tower* (page
206)
½ grapefruit sprinkled with 1 teaspoon of
Flora-Key

Snack
Berry Wonderful Frappé* (page 201)

Lunch
Fresh Tomato Basil Pizza made with 1
Ezekiel 4:9 tortilla, 4 ounces of grilled
chicken, ¼ cup of tomato sauce, tomato slices, and fresh basil leaves. Bake at
425°F for 5 minutes, or until the sauce
is bubbly.

Fat Flush on the Fly: *Plain rotisseried chicken*

Snack
A bowl of veggie broth with sliced green
onions, daikon radish, and cayenne
1 hard-boiled egg

Dinner
4 ounces baked meat loaf made with 1
pound of lean ground beef, 1 egg, ¼
cup of chia seeds, and 2 tablespoons
Fat Flush Seasoning* (page 235). Bake
at 350°F for 40 minutes, or until the
meat loaf has an internal temperature
of 170°F.
½ cup roasted kabocha squash with
ground cumin and 1 tablespoon of
flaxseed oil

Timesaver Tip! *Save 4 ounces of meat loaf for
Day 5's Lunch.*

DAY 4

On Arising
Spiced Lemon Toddy* (page 200)
Green Life Cocktail* (page 199)

Breakfast
Butternut Squashed Fritters* (page 204)

Snack
Zucchini and jicama rounds (raw) with 2
tablespoons of salsa
1 hard-boiled egg

Lunch
Turkey Lettuce Wrap made with 4 ounces
of roasted turkey, Dijon mustard,
chopped cucumber, and shredded carrot, wrapped in a large lettuce leaf
1 serving Artichoke and Hearts of Palm
Salad* (page 230)

Fat Flush on the Fly: *Applegate Farms
Roasted Turkey*

Snack
1 cup raspberries sprinkled with 1 teaspoon of Flora-Key

Dinner
4 ounces oven-roasted yellow snapper rubbed with garlic and ground
coriander
Steamed sugar snap peas and orange bell
pepper with ginger and 1 tablespoon
of lemon-flavored fish oil
½ cup roasted turnips mashed with dill and
1 tablespoon of chia seeds

DAY 5

On Arising
Spiced Lemon Toddy* (page 200)
Green Life Cocktail* (page 199)

Breakfast
Rhubarb-Berry Burst Frappé* (page 202)

Snack
2 hard-boiled eggs with ¼ cup Roasted
Red Pepper Sauce* (page 236)

Lunch
Meat Loaf Burrito made with 4 ounces of
leftover meat loaf, shredded lettuce,
green onions, and 1 warmed Ezekiel
4:9 tortilla, topped with 2 tablespoons
of salsa

Snack
1 Fabulous Chia Crax* (page 246)
1 orange

Dinner
1 serving Pan-Roasted Chicken with Sweet
Potatoes* (page 210)
Steamed mustard greens with lemon and
cayenne

DAY 6

On Arising
Spiced Lemon Toddy* (page 200)
Green Life Cocktail* (page 199)

Breakfast
2 poached eggs
Wilted baby spinach tossed with 1 slice of cooked and crumbled turkey bacon
½ grapefruit sprinkled with 1 teaspoon of Flora-Key

Snack
½ cup Roasted Eggplant Spread* (page 247)
Red, orange, and green pepper wedges

Lunch
Crabmeat Salad made with 4 ounces of crabmeat, chopped red onion, celery, and 2 tablespoons of Fresh Herbed Mayonnaise* (page 235)
Warmed asparagus with freshly squeezed lemon juice
1 slice French Meadow Healthseed Spelt Bread, toasted

Snack
Choco-Cherry Oblivion Frappé* (page 201)

Dinner
4 ounces grilled sirloin with Fat Flush Seasoning* (page 235)
½ cup roasted parsnips with ginger and 1 tablespoon of chia seeds
Steamed broccoli rabe with garlic and basil

DAY 7

On Arising
Spiced Lemon Toddy* (page 200)
Green Life Cocktail* (page 199)

Breakfast
Blueberry Mini Chiacakes* (page 204)

Snack
Bowl of beef broth with snow peas, water chestnuts, and a pinch of Seaweed Gomasio

Lunch
2 cups Cucumber, Wakame, and Tofu Salad* (page 220)
1 Ezekiel 4:9 tortilla, lightly toasted

Snack
1 apple, sliced and sprinkled with 1 tablespoon of chia seeds

Dinner
2 cups Indian Lamb Curry* (page 215)
½ cup steamed garden peas with ground coriander
Oven-roasted spaghetti squash with ginger and 1 tablespoon of flaxseed oil

12 SPRING WELLNESS PROGRAM

SPRING IS A GOOD TIME TO SCHEDULE a routine checkup with your health-care provider and dentist. If any of your winter blood test levels were out of range, repeat the blood work to measure improvement (see resources, page 260).

SPRING BACH FLOWER REMEDY

Spring Fat Flush is a time of renewal and wiping the slate clean. This can also be a time of irritability for many due to the activation of the liver in spring, which is connected with the emotion of anger. Never fear, a Bach Flower Remedy is near: Impatiens. Just as the Bach Flower essence of Oak was used for Winter Fat Flush, Impatiens will support Spring Fat Flush by helping you to achieve tranquility and peace of mind when progress is not as immediate as you would like—especially for those that are in for the long haul with more than fifty pounds to lose.

I suggest that you add four drops of Impatiens to eight ounces of Cranberry H_2O or plain water four times per day and sip it at intervals throughout the day. This remedy restores feelings of inner peace, relaxation, and patience, encouraging you to continue on toward your weight loss and overall wellness goal. For many, Impatiens can take the edge off frustration and upset.

Healing Spring Rituals

■ Record your food, supplements, exercise, and special reflections in a journal.

■ Set aside one day each week to rest, reflect, and regenerate (Sabbath Ritual).

■ Do a thorough spring-cleaning of your home, office or workspace, and car to prepare your psyche for your internal spring cleansing. Decluttering your "outer space" will reduce stress, anxiety, and those feelings of being overwhelmed, allowing you to recharge your "inner space."

■ Make a green sweep by replacing chemical cleaners with natural products such as borox, white vinegar, and baking soda. To kill bacteria, germs, and molds, try distilled white vinegar. To clean metals and plastics and absorb odors and neutralize acids, use baking soda. Use borox as a laundry booster, multipurpose cleaner, and fungicide.

My mental outlook has never been better these past eight years. I feel great and look good. To me, Fat Flush works because it is a lifestyle, not a diet.

—Randall, Fat Flush Fan

ADVANCED SPRING DETOX TECHNIQUES

Do daily **oil pulling** for twenty minutes upon arising.

Castor Oil Pack (3 successive days, 3 days off, then repeat cycle every week or every other week throughout Spring Fat Flush)

The castor oil pack is used to stimulate the liver and gallbladder as well as to draw toxins out of your body. The use of castor oil packs can result in a normalizing of liver enzymes, a decrease in elevated cholesterol levels, and a greater sense of well-being.

Using castor oil packs is as easy as one, two, three. You will need: 100 percent pure, cold-pressed castor oil; wool (not cotton) flannel; and a heating pad. To do the treatment, follow these simple steps:

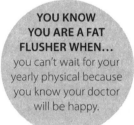

YOU KNOW
YOU ARE A FAT
FLUSHER WHEN…
you can't wait for your
yearly physical because
you know your doctor
will be happy.

1. Fold the wool flannel into three or four layers and soak it with castor oil.
2. Place the soaked flannel in a baking dish and heat it slowly in the oven until it is hot to your touch.
3. Lie down, gently rub 3 tablespoons of castor oil on your abdomen, then place the soaked flannel across your abdomen.
4. Cover the soaked flannel with plastic wrap or plastic garbage bag.
5. Finally, cover the soaked flannel with the heating pad for 1 hour to keep it comfortably hot (but not too hot).

When you finish, wash the oil from your abdomen. You can keep the oil-soaked flannel sealed in plastic wrap or place it in a plastic storage bag for further use, since castor oil does not become rancid as quickly as many other oils.

As a gentle detox, I recommend that you use the castor oil pack once a day for three successive days, take three days off, and then use it for another three days in a row. Continue this pattern weekly or every other week, depending upon your liver enzyme levels. If you suffer from frequent colds, infections, or chronic fatigue syndrome, consider using the castor oil pack on a daily basis for two weeks out of every month while on Spring Fat Flush.

Try a **Manual Lymphatic Drainage** (MLD) massage. Debuting in Paris in the 1930s, this technique is exceedingly gentle with special strokes, stretches, and light, fluttery movements that unclog the lymph system. Check out www.lymphnet.org to find an MLD therapist in your area.

Experience an **ionic footbath**. This new therapy utilizes a very low-intensity current to create a mild electromagnetic field in a mineral and salt bath. If you put your feet into this field, it will help to boost lymphatic flow and fluid exchange. A 20-minute session is all it takes to see a chemical change in the minerals by the ionization process, which often leaves the water looking rather muddy. The color changes that take place during the process are not "toxins" being expelled through the feet but are instead natural changes by the ionization process. The Web sites to check out include www.theionspa.com and www.ionchi.com.

> ### Rejuvenating Spring Mini-Indulgences
>
> ■ Treat yourself to a full day at the spa where you can get a head-to-toe makeover.
> ■ Take time to smell the tulips and daffodils.

Aromatherapy Baths (20 minutes, 3 times a week before bed)

Continue to enjoy aromatherapy baths. You may wish to try different essential oils from those used in Winter Fat Flush. I suggest such oils as Cyprus, which restores skin tone and strengthens weak connective tissue; Orange, which stimulates circulation and continues to help lymphatic flow; and Clary Sage, which supports endocrine function and helps remove fluid from the tissues. You might also try:

■ Rosemary—regenerating, restorative, and detoxifying

■ Lemon—improves clarity of mind and disinfects. (You can also put a few drops in a spray bottle and spray the house for an uplifting, clean scent.)

■ Juniper—promotes toxic waste elimination

■ Lavender—calming and regenerative

You may also apply aromatherapy oils to the soles of your feet in 2 teaspoons of a carrier oil such as almond or jojoba oil, for a detox boost first thing in the morning. By this time, you'll find yourself so serene, energized, and productive, I can't imagine your going back to your old way of life, can you?

13 SPRING FITNESS PLAN

NOW THAT YOU'VE REACHED SPRING and you're reducing your Clean Carb intake, you're going to need to lessen the intensity of your exercise routine as well. But don't worry; you'll still be building lean muscle mass, the most metabolically active tissue in the body, so you'll be burning fat and calories even when you are resting. You'll be less fatigued, your balance and coordination will even be more improved, your flexibility will be increased and, best of all, you'll continue to lose weight because you are still gaining muscle tone. You've already transformed your body composition by increasing your muscle-to-fat ratio. Flushed with success, you are more confident, glowing, and more shapely than ever.

Now that the weather is finally changing, do try to balance your exercise between indoor and outdoor activities. Remember that it is markedly more helpful to exercise in the outdoors for invigorating fresh air and to catch those bone-building, immune-enhancing vitamin D rays. An added bonus is that the sunlight also provides healthy stimulation to the optic nerve, which tones each and every gland of the body.

Enjoy tennis, volleyball, badminton, and low-impact aerobic dancing three to four days a week. Being outside will oxygenate your system and help the cleansing process. For those with very low bone density, concentrate on swimming, walking in water, water aerobics, or cycling rather than on impact activities, which can increase fracture risk.

> Please remember to warm up properly before you begin each workout and cool down with stretching at the end, to lessen soreness and increase flexibility.

Spring Workout Summary

Yoga-Quickies (*5 to 10 minutes, 5 days a week*) *Turn to page 49 in the Pre–Fat Flush Fitness Plan for a description of these moves.*

Cardio Workouts (*35 minutes for Workouts 1 and 2; 20 minutes for Workout 3; 5 days a week, select Workout 1, 2, or 3*)

Workout 1—Walkout for Treadmill

Workout 2—A Walk in the Park

Workout 3—Rebounding

Core Exercises (*5 to 10 minutes, 3 nonconsecutive days a week*)

SPRING CARDIO WORKOUTS

Your goal is to complete 35 minutes of cardio, five days a week. For the sake of variety, I am providing three alternative cardio workout options. Choose which works best for you, keeping in mind that rebounding for 20 minutes is roughly equivalent to 35 minutes of other forms of cardio.

YOU KNOW YOU ARE A FAT FLUSHER WHEN... you go to turn out the lamp and your wedding ring flies across the room.

Cardio Option 1—Walkout for the Treadmill

Duration: 35 minutes; follow the Rate of Perceived Exertion (RPE) scale (see page 57)

Frequency: 5 days a week total cardio options

Targets: Cardiovascular and lymphatic systems

Body-Shaping Tools: Walking shoes

If you have never used a treadmill before you will want to start out slowly at first. It's natural to want to hold on to the handrails initially. As you feel more secure, you will want to pump your arms while walking, to get the lymph moving.

Walkout for the Treadmill Routine

Warm-Up Walk	5 minutes; RPE 3–4
Walk	3 minutes, increase speed to 3.5 mph; RPE 5–6
Walk	3 minutes, increase speed to 3.8 mph; RPE 6–7
Walk	5 minutes, decrease speed to 3 mph; increase incline to 5 (pump your arms as you climb); RPE 7–8
Walk	3 minutes, increase speed to 3.5 mph; decrease incline to 0; RPE 3–4
Walk	5 minutes; decrease speed to 2.6 mph; increase incline to 10 (pump your arms as you climb); RPE 8–9
Walk	3 minutes; increase speed to 3.5 mph; decrease incline to 0; RPE 5–6
Walk	3 minutes; increase speed to 3.8 mph; RPE 6–7
Cool-Down Walk	5 minutes; RPE 3–4

Total Workout Time: 35 minutes, including warm-up and cool-down.

Cardio Option 2—A Walk in the Park Interval Training

Duration: 35 minutes; follow instructions for each segment as indicated
Frequency: 5 days a week
Targets: Cardiovascular and lymphatic systems and full body toning
Body-Shaping Tools: Walking shoes

This routine combines cardio interval training with toning. It is an outdoor workout that will blast you into shape and you won't even have to step foot in the gym.

Turn to page 93 in Winter Fat Flush for a description of these moves.

Warm-Up Segment—Walking
Duration: 5 minutes; RPE 1–3

Cardio Toning Segment 1—Alternating Lunges
Duration: 1 minute; RPE 5–6

> "Maintaining aerobic fitness through middle age and beyond can delay biological aging by up to 12 years and prolong independence during old age," concludes an analysis published in the *British Journal of Sports Medicine.*[1]

Cardio Segment 1—Walking
Duration: 5 minutes; RPE 3–4

Cardio Toning Segment 2—Park Bench Push-ups
Duration: 1 minute; 12 to 15 repetitions; RPE 5–6

Cardio Segment 2—Walking
Duration: 5 minutes; RPE 4–5

Cardio Toning Segment 3—Side Lunges
Duration: 1 minute; 12 to 15 repetitions; RPE 5–6

Cardio Segment 3—Speed Walk or Run
Duration: 5 minutes; RPE 6–7

Cardio Toning Segment 4—Park Bench Dips
Duration: 1 minute; 12 to 15 repetitions; RPE 5–6
Body-Shaping Tool: Bench

Cardio Segment 4—Speed Walk or Run
Duration: 5 minutes; RPE 6–7

Cardio Toning Segment 5—Skipping
Duration: 1 minute; RPE 5–6

Cool-Down Segment
Duration: 5 minutes; RPE 1–3
Walk at a slower pace to bring your heart rate to the cool-down stretch levels.
Total Workout Time: 35 minutes, includes warm-up and cool-down

Cardio Option 3—Rebounding
Duration: 20 minutes (to the beat of your favorite iPod tunes)
Frequency: 5 days a week
Targets: Cardiovascular and lymphatic systems
Body-Shaping Tool: Rebounder
Two new upper-body exercises—the Shoulder Press and the Chest Press—are added to a more intense bouncing routine for an advanced workout.
Start to jog on the rebounder. With your arms at shoulder height, do a shoulder press, then do a chest press. Continue to jog and alternate between the shoulder press and chest press.

Moderate Jog with Shoulder Press
Jog on your rebounder at a light but moderate pace. Start with both arms bent, at your sides and your hands at shoulder level. Press and straighten your arms upward. Then lower your arms back down to shoulder level starting position. Continue to jog while repeating this motion.

Moderate Jog with Chest Press
Jog on your rebounder at a light but moderate pace. Start with both arms bent, at your sides and your hands at chest level. Press and straighten your arms forward. Then bring them back toward your chest. Continue to job while repeating this motion.

Spring Rebounding Routine
Warm-up Light Bounce—3 minutes
Cardio Phase—14 minutes
Moderate Bounce—2 minutes
Moderate Bounce or Jog with Chest Press—2 minutes
Moderate Bounce or Jog with Shoulder Press—2 minutes

Moderate Jog—2 minutes

Moderate Bounce or Jog with Combined Chest and Shoulder Press—2 minutes

Heel-Jack Bounce—2 minutes

Jumping Jack Bounce—2minutes

Cool-Down Light Bounce—3 minutes

Total Workout Time: 20 minutes, including warm-up and cool-down

CORE EXERCISES

Medicine Ball Crunch

Duration: 1 set of 10

Frequency: 3 nonconsecutive days per week

Torso Twist

Duration: 1 set of 10; do set 3 times

Frequency: 3 nonconsecutive days per week

Side Plank

Duration: 1 set of 10; do set 3 times

Frequency: 3 nonconsecutive days per week

Back Extension

Duration: 1 set of 10; do set 3 times

Frequency: 3 days per week total

Turn to page 97 in the Winter Fitness Plan for a full description of each of these moves.

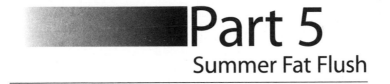

Part 5

Summer Fat Flush

14 SUMMER FAT FLUSH DIET

You cannot turn back the clock. But you can wind it up again.

—*Bonnie Prudden*

THERE IS A LUXURIOUS AND LUSH QUALITY about the summer season. Nature is in full bloom and the stage is set for vitality and maturation. Your body's innate wisdom is preparing your system for more activity, which in turn, highly energizes your heart. This fired-up season lends itself to a focus on your heart and small intestine, the organs most vulnerable in summer. Seasonal symptoms related to these organs include:

- Angina, shortness of breath
- Slow, irregular pulse
- Numbness or tingling, generally in the left arm or hand
- Constipation or diarrhea
- Bloating, belching, embarrassing flatulence
- Heartburn
- Tiredness after eating
- Halitosis

To support these vital organs through the heat of summer, Summer Fat Flush features a larger selection of juicy fresh fruits and fiber-rich veggies in salads that are loaded with enzymes to enhance digestion, increase elimination, and help cool off summer heat from the body. Tomatoes, fresh off the vine, offer heart

Teas and Herbs that Cleanse, Heal, and Relax

Rose Hips tea is the summertime tea of choice, which is very refreshing as iced tea. Go ahead and drink one to two cups a day if you have any of the symptoms that relate to the heart and small intestine. It provides a rich supply of vitamin C, which supports the heart, blood vessels, immune system, and lining of the GI tract.

Heart- and GI tract–protecting herbs include: hawthorn berries, which can normalize blood pressure and treat angina and irregular heartbeat; licorice root, which reduces inflammation and cleanses the intestinal tract; cayenne, which helps to regulate circulation and stimulate the heart; and garlic, summer's stinking rose, which is an antibacterial, to protect pathogens in the intestinal tract and to heal mucosal membranes while revving up circulation.

healthy potassium, vitamin B$_6$, and folic acid as well as the phytonutrient lyco-pene, to enhance overall health and quench summer palates.

Summer also happens to be the ideal time to do an extreme detox. Summer Fat Flush begins with an accelerated 14-day diet that flushes accumulated toxins from the lymphatic system and from your stores of fat and jump-starts weight loss. You can extend the fourteen-day cleanse an additional two weeks, especially if you have more than 25 pounds to lose or want to maintain a clean and healthy detox and diet for summer. Most individuals lose weight extremely quickly dur-ing this phase. Many who have lots of weight to lose have reported a loss of up to a pound a day and as many as twelve inches.

Just be prepared.

This is a time when many individuals can feel initially tired, especially those who are just beginning Fat Flush for Life and starting with Summer as they give up their multiple cups of coffee, sugar, and grains that have been providing them with quick fixes of temporary energy. Some can even experience headaches, nau-sea, and other types of discomfort as they withdraw from their reliance on coffee and "high blood sugar" foods or as their bodies respond to the toxins that are being released from the systems. But this lasts only for a short period of time (about four days, to be exact)—and then they begin to feel almost euphoric.

The irony here is although Summer Fat Flush is extreme with regard to the diet, this is *not* the time to engage in extreme exercise. On the contrary, this is a time to take it easy. You are not going to be eating enough carbs—at least in the first two to four weeks—that are necessary for strenuous physical exercise and weight training. Therefore the Summer Fitness Plan has been adjusted accordingly. But, no worries, your body will readjust and allow you to engage in more vigorous workouts again once the accelerated detox portion of Summer Fat Flush is over.

Another key to the high success rate has always been the food itself—yes, even during the extreme detox weeks. Many people are fascinated with a detox pro-gram that allows you to enjoy quick and easy gourmet meals such as Crab Cakes in a Flash and a decadent array of frappés such as Raspberry Truffle and Black-berry Blast, which taste like desserts.

In the accelerated part of the plan, some foods will continue to be temporarily eliminated. These include dairy (except whey protein, which does not contain the allergens casein and lactose of regular milk products), including cheese, starchy vegetables, and grains—other than the sprouted grains in the Fat Flush–legal bread and tortilla group. Most grains, but especially the gluten-containing ones such as wheat, rye, and barley, can be allergenic to nearly 50 percent of the popu-lation, creating an inflammatory response that can result in five to ten pounds of water retention.

After you complete the extreme detox portion of Summer Fat Flush (two to four weeks), you may continue to enjoy all these deliciously satisfying foods while slowly adding back up to two "lighter" Clean Carb selections for the remainder of the summer. Start with one selection per day for at least two weeks and then increase to one and a half Clean Carbs for another two weeks until you are able to tolerate two Clean Carbs without any bloating, fatigue, or weight gain. Selections can include ½ cup of fresh green peas or cooked carrots, quinoa, oats, Ezekiel 4:9 sprouted-grain tortillas, and French Meadow Healthseed Spelt Bread.

For some very sensitive individuals, even the sprouted grain–based carbs can trigger food sensitivity reactions, which may be delayed by a couple of hours or even days after eating. If bloating starts, sinuses act up, and weight loss stalls, this may be a sign of a toxic food reaction. You need to scale back or eliminate these foods immediately while substituting a more body-friendly Clean Carb.

Follow Extreme Summer Fat Flush for two to four weeks. By filling up on the program's nutrient-packed foods, you'll feel more energetic and your skin will look smoother and sleeker. You will even lose lots of weight—in as little as two weeks' time.

> *The first thing I noticed was a big smoothing out of cellulite. My sense is that my body began using the better nutrients to work from the inside out.*
>
> —*Fat Flush online fan*

SUMMER FAT FLUSHING SUPERSTAR FOODS

Following, you will find delicious and nutritious options to integrate into the Fat Flush menus and recipes, including a wonderful expanded list of cooling, refreshing, detoxifying in-season fruits. Use these to widen your variety of healthy food choices for lifelong weight control, long-term satiety, and well-being. PS: You will love wearing out those "skinny jeans"!

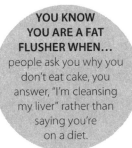

YOU KNOW YOU ARE A FAT FLUSHER WHEN... people ask you why you don't eat cake, you answer, "I'm cleansing my liver" rather than saying you're on a diet.

Cranberry H$_2$O
Recipe: See page 198.
Bodily Consumption: 64 ounces per day between each meal and snack, in Green Life Cocktail, and in frappés.

Hot Lemon Water

Benefits: This is your Hot Lemon Toddy from the Winter Fat Flush, sans
cinnamon and ginger.
Recipe: See page 200.
Bodily Consumption: Daily on arising

Green Life Cocktail

Recipe: See page 199.
Bodily Consumption: Daily on arising

Probiotic Sweetener

Benefits: Contains beneficial bacteria to balance GI tract for weight-loss insurance
and enhanced immunity. Provides yeast-free sweetener for no-heat frappés,
beverages, and desserts.
Brands: UNI KEY's Flora-Key
Bodily Consumption: 2 to 3 teaspoons per day in Green Life Cocktails and frappés,
and with nonheated foods

Whey Protein

Benefits: Assists lean muscle mass development, increases energy, natural appetite
suppressant
Brands: UNI KEY's Fat Flush Vanilla or Chocolate Whey Protein
Bodily Consumption: Up to 2 servings per day (20 grams protein each) in frappés,
muffins, desserts, whey pancakes, etc. *Note:* Chocolate whey is limited to 2
servings per week.

Chia Seeds

Bodily Consumption: 2 to 3 tablespoons per day, added to frappés, soups, stews,
and dressings or sprinkled on such foods as eggs and veggies

Slimming Oils

Choose from:
High-lignan Flaxseed Oil
Bodily Consumption: Total of two tablespoons per day of flaxseed oil and/or fish
oil. Do not heat flaxseed oil.

Fish Oil
Bodily Consumption: Total of 2 tablespoons per day of flaxseed oil and/or fish oil.
Do not heat fish oil.

Extra-Virgin Olive Oil in an oil mister (such as Misto).
Bodily Consumption: Lightly spritz in cooking as needed.

Herbs, Spices, and Seasonings
Choose from:

Anise

Apple cider vinegar

Bay leaves (fresh or dried)

Cayenne

Chives (fresh or dried)

Cilantro

Cinnamon

Cloves

Coriander

Cream of tartar

Cumin

Dill (fresh or dried)

Dry mustard

Fennel (fresh or dried)

Garlic (fresh or garlic powder)

Ginger (fresh or dried)

Mint (fresh or dried)

Onion powder

Parsley (fresh or dried)

Turmeric

Wasabi

Bodily Consumption: ¼ to ½ teaspoon at least 3 to 5 times per week

Protein
Bodily Consumption: a minimum of 8 ounces of cooked lean protein
Choose from:

Suggested varieties of canned or fresh fish, shellfish, and seafood (wild encouraged)

Lean beef, lamb, veal (organic/grass-fed encouraged), and other meats

Poultry

Omega-enriched eggs (hormone-free/free-range encouraged)

Vegetarian Protein Sources: Tofu and tempeh

Fish
Choose from:
Fresh

Bass

Cod

Grouper

Haddock

Halibut

Mackerel

Mahimahi

Orange roughy

Perch

Pike

Pollock

Salmon

Sardines

Snapper

Sole

Squid

Trout

Tuna

Whitefish

Canned

Crabmeat

(Featherweight,

Seasons, Lillie, Three

Star)

Light tuna—not

| albacore (Natural Sea, Crown Prince) Mackerel Salmon (Natural Sea, Crown Prince, Vital Choice) | Sardines (Bela, Olhao, Crown Prince) *Shellfish* Calamari | Crab Lobster Scallops Shrimp |

Meat
Choose from:
Lean beef, lamb, veal, and other meats

Look for free-range, grass-fed lean meat found in health food stores or supermarkets or online companies such as Niman Ranch (www.nimanranch.com). My personal favorite is Ranch Foods Direct (www.ranchfoodsdirect.com), a specialty meat company selling natural beef, raised without hormones or antibiotics. This company combines the best of traditional animal husbandry practices with an innovative processing method.

Beef	*Lamb*	*Other Meats*
Brisket	Leg	Elk
Chuck	Loin	Ostrich
Eye of round	Rib	Venison
Flank		Bison from Hole
London broil	*Veal*	Buffalo Company
Round	Loin	(www.jhbuffalomeat
Rump	Rib	.com) and Buffalo
Sirloin	Shoulder	Gal (www.buffalogal .com)

Poultry
Choose from:
White meat of skinned turkey and chicken, fresh or frozen. Look for free-range and hormone-free, such as Foster Farms, Harmony Farms, Shelton Farms, and Young Farms.

In addition to the above protein choices you may also enjoy:

Omega-Enriched Eggs
Bodily Consumption: Up to 2 per day

Vegetarian Protein Sources

Choose from:

Tofu—unflavored, firm and silken (Mori-Nu, White Wave)

Tempeh (Turtle Island Foods, Lightlife)

Bodily Consumption: Up to 2 servings (4 ounces each) of tofu and/or tempeh per week

Fruits

Benefits: The following healthy fruits offer collagen-enhancing vitamin C and enzyme-activating potassium, and they help maintain balanced blood sugar.

Brands (frozen): Frozen fruits are acceptable as well, such as Woodstock Farms (www.woodstock-farms.com), Cascadian Farm (www.cfarm.com), and Stahlbush Farm (www.stahlbush.com).

Bodily Consumption: Up to 2 servings per day

Choose from:

1 small apple, orange, nectarine, peach, pear, or pomegranate

1 cup berries (blueberries, blackberries, raspberries, and/or cranberries)

6 large strawberries

10 large cherries

2 medium-size plums

½ grapefruit

Lemons and limes (as desired)

½ cup grapes

½ cup pineapple

1 cup melon (watermelon, cantaloupe, and honeydew)

2 kiwis

1 small banana

Vegetables

Fresh: Look for fresh (in season locally is best) vegetables that are full of vibrant color so that you can eat the rainbow.

Brands (frozen): Frozen vegetables are acceptable as well, such as Woodstock Farms (www.woodstock-farms.com), Cascadian Farm (www.cfarm.com), and Stahlbush Farm (www.stahlbush.com).

Brands (canned): No added salt or sugar

Bodily Consumption: Aim for at least 5 or more servings per day.

A vegetable serving is generally 1 cup raw or ½ cup cooked

Choose from:

(All unlimited except where noted)

Artichokes (1 whole or 5 hearts)
Arugula
Asparagus
Bamboo shoots
Bell peppers (red, green, and orange)
Bok choy
Broccoli
Brussels sprouts
Burdock
Cabbage
Carrots (limit 1 medium-size or 5 baby)
Cauliflower
Celery
Celery root
Chard
Chinese cabbage
Chives
Cilantro
Collard greens
Cucumbers
Daikon
Dandelion greens

Eggplant
Endive
Escarole
Green beans
Hearts of palm
Jalapeños
Jerusalem artichoke
Jicama
Kale
Kohlrabi
Leeks
Lettuce (red or green, romaine, butter, baby greens, etc.)
Mushrooms
Mustard greens
Okra
Olives (black, 3 per day)
Onions
Parsley
Radicchio
Radishes
Rhubarb (1 cup)
Shallots
Snow peas
Spaghetti squash

Spinach
Sprouts (alfalfa, mung bean, broccoli)
Sugar snap peas
Tomatillos
Tomatoes and tomato products (see below)
Water chestnuts
Watercress
Yellow squash
Zucchini

Tomato Products (no added sugar or salt)
Diced tomatoes
Pizza sauce
Tomato paste
Tomato puree
Tomato sauce
Whole peeled tomatoes
Brands: Muir Glen, Eden, Bio Nature, Woodstock Farms

Sea Vegetables

Benefits: Rich in iodine and many trace minerals such as calcium and iron, sea veggies support thyroid function and also inhibit the absorption of radiation and heavy metals.

Choose from: Agar, arame, hijiki, kombu, nori, sea palm fronds, wakame

Brand: Eden

Bodily Consumption: Up to 2 servings of 1 tablespoon agar and/or ½ cup of arame, hijiki, kombu, nori, sea palm fronds, and wakame per week added to soups, stews, poultry, beef, fish, seafood, salads, veggies, eggs, etc.
You may also add a sea veggie–based seasoning:
Brand: Eden Seaweed Gomasio (contains sea vegetables, sesame seeds, and sea salt)
Bodily Consumption: ½ teaspoon daily

Beverages

Healing Tea
Rose hips tea
Brands: Alvita, Traditional Medicinals
Bodily Consumption: 1 to 2 cups per day

Legal Cheats

Organic coffee (caffeinated)
Benefits: Provides antioxidants and B vitamins such as niacin
Brands: Newman's Own Organics, Organic Coffee Co.
Bodily Consumption: 1 cup each day

Salt
Brands: Morton's Canning and Pickling Salt, Real Salt, Himalayan Pink Salt

Bodily Consumption: ½ to 1 teaspoon per day (Use your best judgment— if you bloat, are hypertensive, or take a diuretic then take less. If you have low blood pressure or suffer from adrenal exhaustion, you can use up to 1 teaspoon per day)

Stevia Plus (for use in heated foods)
Bodily Consumption: Maximum of 2 (0.035-ounce or 1-gram) packets per day

A GENTLE REMINDER—ESPECIALLY FOR SUMMER FAT FLUSH

- Menu plans are completely optional. If following a structured plan is not for you, feel free to create your own fabulous Fat Flush–friendly meals and snacks that follow the Summer Fat Flush guidelines.
- Recipes noted with an asterisk (*) are found in chapter 21.
- Lunches, dinners, and snacks are interchangeable within the same day.
- You may add an extra tablespoon of chia seeds into recipes, if desired.
- Make sure to drink a total of 64 ounces of Cranberry H_2O daily between meals. Eight ounces of Cranberry H_2O are included in a once daily Green Life Cocktail. You may also drink as much plain filtered water as you would like, provided you have consumed the recommended 64 ounces of Cranberry H_2O. In addition, one cup of organic coffee and one to two rose hips tea per day is also acceptable.
- Continue to maintain your results with the Fat Flush Kit supplements: the Dieters' Multi (with or without iron) for balanced vitamin and mineral supplementation; the GLA 90s for stimulating brown adipose tissue metabolism, which increases fat burning and keeps skin moist and taut during weight loss; and the Weight Loss Formula for carbohydrate control, fat metabolism and liver support (without stimulants). Also continue to take 1,000 mg of CLA three times per day with meals.

SUMMER FAT FLUSH EXTREME DETOX: 14-DAY MEAL PLANNER

DAY 1

On Arising
Hot Lemon Water* (page 200)
Green Life Cocktail* (page 199)

Breakfast
Blackberry Blast Frappé* (page 201)

Snack
2 hard-boiled eggs with Fat Flush Seasoning* (page 235)
Zucchini and jicama rounds (raw)

Fat Flush on the Fly: Look for Eggland's Best Hard-Cooked Peeled Eggs

Lunch
Roast Beef and Veggie Lettuce Wraps

made with 4 ounces of roast beef, veggies, and 2 tablespoons of E-Z Classic Mayo* (page 235), wrapped in large lettuce leaves

Fat Flush on the Fly: Applegate Farms Roast Beef Slices

Snack
6 large strawberries sprinkled with 1 teaspoon of Flora-Key

Dinner
4 ounces grilled mahi mahi with lemon and Seaweed Gomasio
Oven-roasted tomato halves with parsley and 1 tablespoon of chia seeds

DAY 2

On Arising
Hot Lemon Water* (page 200)
Green Life Cocktail* (page 199)

Breakfast
2 poached eggs on bed of steamed
arugula
1 cup blueberries

Snack
Just Cherries Frappé* (page 201)

Lunch
4 ounces canned salmon with celery and
parsley
2 tablespoons E-Z Classic Mayo* (page 235)
Leafy green salad

Fat Flush on the Fly: *No time to make
homemade mayo? Try 1 tablespoon of
Spectrum's Organic Omega-3 Mayonnaise with Flax Oil.*

Snack
Sliced cucumbers with apple cider vinegar
and dill

Dinner
2 cups 1-2-3 Salsa Chicken* (page 209)
Wilted baby spinach with lemon, garlic,
and 1 tablespoon of chia seeds

Timesaver Tips! *Start your slow cooker before
you leave in the morning so dinner will be
just about ready when you come home!
Save leftover chicken and prepare some
extra spinach for Day 3's Lunch.*

DAY 3

On Arising
Hot Lemon Water* (page 200)
Green Life Cocktail* (page 199)

Breakfast
Raspberry Truffle Frappé* (page 202)

Snack
2 hard-boiled eggs with Seaweed Gomasio
Broccoli and cauliflower florets

Lunch
2 cups leftover 1-2 3 Salsa Chicken*
Leftover steamed spinach with lemon and
garlic

Snack
½ cup grapes

Dinner
4 ounces broiled veal chop with Fat Flush
Seasoning* (page 235)
Steamed green beans with garlic, cilantro,
and 1 tablespoon of chia seeds
Baby greens, grated carrot, and broccoli
sprouts salad with apple cider vinegar
and 1 tablespoon of flaxseed oil

DAY 4

On Arising
Hot Lemon Water* (page 200)
Green Life Cocktail* (page 199)

Breakfast
2 scrambled eggs with bell peppers and a pinch of Fat Flush Seasoning* (page 235)
½ grapefruit sprinkled with 1 teaspoon of Flora-Key

Snack
A bowl of chicken broth with diced veggies, cayenne, and 1 tablespoon of chia seeds

Fat Flush on the Fly: Imagine Free-Range Chicken Broth

Lunch
Simple Tuna Salad made with 4 ounces of canned tuna, celery, peppers, broccoli sprouts, and 2 tablespoons of E-Z Fat Flush Vinaigrette* (page 237)
Mixed baby greens

Snack
Blushing Peach Frappé* (page 201)

Dinner
Tofu Veggie Stir-fry made with 4 ounces of tofu, plus water chestnuts, mushrooms, snow peas, and garlic, stir-fried in veggie broth
Steamed cabbage with Seaweed Gomasio and a splash of apple cider vinegar

DAY 5

On Arising
Hot Lemon Water* (page 200)
Green Life Cocktail* (page 199)

Breakfast
Berry Wonderful Frappé* (page 201)

Snack
Cherry tomatoes and freshly squeezed lime juice
1 hard-boiled egg with Seaweed Gomasio

Lunch
Shrimp Salad made with 4 ounces of cooked shrimp, plus celery, red onion, and 2 tablespoons of Fresh Herbed Mayonnaise* (page 235)
Romaine lettuce "scoopers"

Fat Flush on the Fly: Look for fresh or frozen precooked shrimp.

Snack
2 plums
1 hard-boiled egg with dry mustard

Dinner
2 cups Turkey Scaloppine Skillet Supper* (page 211)
Steamed spaghetti squash with coriander and 1 tablespoon of chia seeds

Timesaver Tip! Save leftover turkey and spaghetti squash for Day 6's Lunch.

DAY 6

On Arising
  Hot Lemon Water* (page 200)
  Green Life Cocktail* (page 199)

Breakfast
  Sunburst Omelet with two eggs, tomato,
    green onion, and cumin
  2 kiwis

Snack
  ½ cup Chunky Artichoke Dip* (page 247)
  Sugar snap peas and red pepper sticks

Lunch
  2 cups leftover Turkey Scaloppine Skillet
    Supper*
  Leftover steamed spaghetti squash with
    parsley

Snack
  Choco-Cherry Oblivion Frappé* (page 201)

Dinner
  2 cups Effortless Beef Chili* (page 212)
    mixed with 1 tablespoon of chia seeds
  Mashed steamed cauliflower with fennel
    and a pinch of cayenne

Timesaver Tips! *Start your slow cooker before
  you leave in the morning so dinner will be
  just about ready when you come home!
  Save leftover chili and prepare extra cauliflower for Day 7's Lunch.*

DAY 7

On Arising
  Hot Lemon Water* (page 200)
  Green Life Cocktail* (page 199)

Breakfast
  Rhubarb-Berry Burst Frappé* (page 202)

Snack
  2 hard-boiled eggs smashed with Seaweed
    Gomasio and 2 tablespoons of E-Z Clas-
    sic Mayo* (page 235)

Lunch
  2 cups leftover Effortless Beef Chili* mixed
    with 1 tablespoon of chia seeds
  Leftover mashed steamed cauliflower

Snack
  1 small banana

Dinner
  4 ounces grilled scallops with lime and Fat
    Flush Seasoning* (page 235)
  Steamed chard with garlic
  Endive salad with artichokes, hearts of
    palm, dill, and a splash of apple cider
    vinegar

DAY 8

On Arising
Hot Lemon Water* (page 200)
Green Life Cocktail* (page 199)

Breakfast
2-egg omelet with baby spinach, a pinch
of cayenne, and 1 tablespoon of chia
seeds
6 large strawberries sprinkled with 1 teaspoon of Flora-Key

Snack
Yellow squash and zucchini rounds (raw)
with 2 tablespoons of salsa

*Fat Flush on the Fly: Muir Glen or Seeds of
Change Salsa*

Lunch
Salmon Salad Lettuce Wraps made with
4 ounces of canned salmon mixed
with 2 tablespoons of Fresh Herbed

Mayonnaise* (page 235), topped with
green onions and broccoli sprouts, and
wrapped in large lettuce leaves

*Fat Flush on the Fly: No time to make
homemade mayo? Try 1 tablespoon of
Spectrum's Omega-3 Organic Mayonnaise with Flax Oil.*

Snack
Pears 'n' Cinnamon Frappé* (page 202)

Dinner
2 cups Cuban Ropa Vieja* (page 212)
Steamed broccolini with lemon and
cilantro
Oven-roasted spaghetti squash with garlic

*Timesaver Tip! Save leftover Cuban Ropa
Vieja and spaghetti squash and prepare
extra broccolini for Day 9's Lunch.*

DAY 9

On Arising
Hot Lemon Water* (page 200)
Green Life Cocktail* (page 199)

Breakfast
2 scrambled eggs with cilantro and a pinch
of Seaweed Gomasio
½ cup cantaloupe sprinkled with 1 teaspoon of Flora-Key

Snack
2 cups Just Vegg 'n-Out Munchies* (page
248)

Lunch
2 cups leftover Cuban Ropa Vieja*
Leftover spaghetti squash and broccolini
with 1 tablespoon of chia seeds

Snack
Choco-Rhuberry Frappé* (page 202)

Dinner
4 ounces grilled halibut with freshly
squeezed lime juice and Fat Flush Seasoning* (page 235)
Baby bok choy steamed in veggie broth
with ginger

DAY 10

On Arising
Hot Lemon Water* (page 200)
Green Life Cocktail* (page 199)

Breakfast
Berry Wonderful Frappé* (page 201)

Snack
2 hard-boiled eggs with pinch of Fat Flush
    Seasoning* (page 235)
Cucumber slices and 5 baby carrots

Fat Flush on the Fly: *Eggland's Best Hard-Cooked Peeled Eggs*

Lunch
2 cups Survival Soup* (page 232)
Baby lettuce, parsley, and cilantro salad
    with 2 tablespoons of Amazing Caesar
    Dressing* (page 237)

Snack
1 nectarine

Dinner
2 Crab Cakes in a Flash* (page 216)
Steamed chard with garlic, lemon, and
    1 tablespoon of chia seeds

Timesaver Tip! *Save 2 crab cakes for Day 11's Lunch.*

DAY 11

On Arising
Hot Lemon Water* (page 200)
Green Life Cocktail* (page 199)

Breakfast
2 poached eggs on a bed of steamed kale
    with a pinch of cumin and 1 table-
    spoon of chia seeds
1 orange

Snack
Cherry tomatoes and 3 artichoke hearts
    with freshly squeezed lime juice and
    parsley

Lunch
2 leftover Crab Cakes in a Flash*
Green beans sautéed in veggie broth and
    coriander

Snack
Blueberry Frappé with a Twist* (page 202)

Dinner
4 ounces grilled lamb burger
Oven-roasted Brussels sprouts with lemon
    drizzled with 1 tablespoon of flaxseed
    oil

Timesaver Tip! *Grill an extra lamb burger and prepare extra Brussels sprouts for Day 12's Lunch.*

DAY 12

On Arising
Hot Lemon Water* (page 200)
Green Life Cocktail* (page 199)

Breakfast
Peaches 'n' Cream Frappé* (page 202)

Snack
Snappy Egg Salad made with 2 hard-boiled
eggs mashed with 2 tablespoons of E-Z
Classic Mayo* (page 235), celery, tur-
meric, and a pinch of cayenne
Snow pea and yellow squash dippers

Fat Flush on the Fly: *No time to make
homemade mayo? Try 1 tablespoon of
Spectrum's Organic Omega-3 Mayonnaise with Flax Oil.*

Lunch
4 ounces leftover lamb burger with Brussels sprouts
Escarole and watercress salad with daikon
radish and 1 tablespoon of apple cider
vinegar

Snack
1 apple

Dinner
4 ounces grilled tilapia with freshly
squeezed lime juice, garlic, and cilantro
Steamed zucchini with ginger and 1 tablespoon of chia seeds

DAY 13

On Arising
Hot Lemon Water* (page 200)
Green Life Cocktail* (page 199)

Breakfast
2 scrambled eggs with parsley and a pinch
of Seaweed Gomasio
½ cup pineapple sprinkled with 1 teaspoon
of Flora-Key

Snack
Berries 'n' Cherries Frappé* (page 202)

Lunch
2 cups Survival Soup* (page 232) mixed
with 1 tablespoon of chia seeds
Butter lettuce salad with grated jicama,
radishes, and 1 tablespoon each of
freshly squeezed lime juice and flaxseed oil

Snack
Sugar snap peas and red pepper rings
3 black olives

Dinner
4 ounces roasted chicken breast with
lemon and Fat Flush Seasoning* (page
235) Wilted Red Cabbage with Fennel*
(page 227)

Fat Flush on the Fly: *Plain rotisseried chicken*

Timesaver Tip! *Roast an extra chicken breast
for Day 14's Lunch*

DAY 14

On Arising
Hot Lemon Water* (page 200)
Green Life Cocktail* (page 199)

Breakfast
Tofu Veggie Scrambler made with 4 ounces of firm tofu scrambled with baby
spinach, bell pepper, 1 tablespoon of
chia seeds, and a pinch of Seaweed
Gomasio
1 orange

Snack
A bowl of veggie broth with green onions
and sliced mushrooms
2 hard-boiled eggs with dry mustard

Lunch
4 ounces leftover roasted chicken
Wilted curly endive with grated carrot,
mung bean sprouts, and 1 tablespoon
each of flaxseed oil and apple cider
vinegar

Snack
Raspberry Truffle Frappé* (page 202)

Dinner
4 ounces grilled beef burger with bell pepper, red onion, lettuce, and tomato
slices
Steamed artichoke with dill and lemon

*Fat Flush on the Fly: Applegate Farms 100%
Beef*

15 SUMMER WELLNESS PROGRAM

THROUGH THE PRECEDING SEASONS, you've been proactive to ensure the healthy functioning of your liver. Since hormones are metabolized by the liver, I now recommend a salivary hormone test to assess hormonal levels, especially estrogen and progesterone, which can impact weight loss big time. While much attention has been paid to the role of estrogen, the importance of progesterone is often overlooked. One of the body's most important hormones, it helps burn body fat for fuel, as opposed to estrogen, which promotes water retention. By making sure our progesterone levels are adequate, we can avoid many of the symptoms of aging. Progesterone stabilizes blood sugar, builds bones, supports the thyroid, it's a diuretic and an antidepressant, helps prevent breast and uterine cancer, and stabilizes the zinc-copper balance in the body. Unlike the traditional blood test, the salivary test accurately measures the levels of hormones that are fully active, known as bioavailable or free.

Blood hormone tests, on the other hand, measure hormones that are 90 to 99 percent bound. Wrapped in protein so they can be transported through the bloodstream, bound hormones are not fully biologically active. Using a blood test to assess hormones gives you and your health practitioner a distorted picture of your biologically active hormone levels.

Healing Summer Rituals

- Record your food, supplements, exercise, and special reflections in a journal.
- Set aside one day each week to rest, reflect, and regenerate (Sabbath Ritual).
- Protect your system with a more *potent probiotic* that can ward off food-born illnesses that are more prevalent during summertime travel. I recommend Dr. Ohhira's Probiotics 12 Plus, which is enteric coated, has proven adhesion; sticks to the walls of the digestive tract for full effectiveness; and is safe for all ages of children, women, and men. And best of all, it does not require refrigeration. You take five in the morning and five at night until you finish one box, then take one in the morning and one at night thereafter, always on an empty stomach. If you do pick up a bug on your travels, then go back to the five in the morning and five at night restorative dosage until symptoms abate. (See resources, page 257.)

A salivary hormone test can be done at home to test for up to six hormones (progesterone, estradiol, estriol, testosterone, DHEA, and cortisol). (See resources, page 257.) This will not only help you tailor your program to address specific hormonal challenges, but it will also give you a baseline to track your results as you progress through *Fat Flush for Life*.

SUMMER BACH FLOWER REMEDY

Summer Fat Flush is the time when many individuals can feel unusually tired as they give up such stimulants as caffeine, sugar, and refined carbs that have been giving them quick bursts of energy. This is why I recommend the Bach Flower Remedy Olive for summer use, which can help overcome exhaustion and physical fatigue.

YOU KNOW YOU ARE A FAT FLUSHER WHEN... you can't go to bed without making a fresh batch of Cranberry H_2O and getting all of your supplements together for the next day.

I suggest that you add four drops of Olive to eight ounces of plain filtered water four times per day and sip it at intervals throughout the day. Remember, you can also put this on your skin or in your bath in the same amounts.

> *I had so much fun preparing the meals and feeling stronger, more*
> *emotionally stable, and my late-night cravings completely stopped!*
> *For the first time ever in my life I had control over my body, mind,*
> *and emotions because I was giving my body proper nutrients.*
>
> —*Emily Jean, Fat Flush Fan*

ADVANCED SUMMER DETOX TECHNIQUES

Do daily **oil pulling** for 10 to 15 minutes upon arising.

Dry Skin Brush Massage (5 minutes, every other day)

The dry skin brush massage is one of my favorite advanced detox techniques. This technique helps you achieve your weight loss goal by stimulating lymph flow, increasing circulation, and stimulating your skin's oil-producing glands. Skin brushing can dramatically help in reducing the appearance of cellulite, rebuilding strong connective tissue, and promoting toned skin, especially important as you continue to lose weight.

Dry brushing is best done early in the day. Plan enough time to take a shower or a relaxing bath after dry brushing because you will want to wash off the dead skin. Do not brush the sensitive skin on your face and of course avoid any areas that are bruised or irritated. Follow these simple steps and remember to always brush toward the heart. Dry brushing will leave your skin glowing and your body feeling invigorated.

- Use a medium-firm vegetable brush with natural bristles (can be purchased in health food store) that is as large as your hand and has a long enough handle to reach your back.
- Start by opening the primary lymph ducts (just below your collarbone and on the right and left groin areas) with a gentle finger massage. Next, begin to brush the soles of your feet vigorously in a circular motion. The amount of pressure depends on the condition of your skin. Using short upward strokes (toward your heart), slowly move up over your feet and legs. Continue up over your abdomen and over your buttocks to your waist.
- Move to the palms of your hands using circular motions, then use short strokes up your hands and arms. Continue brushing down your neck—out to your shoulders and then down your chest and your back.
- This can be followed with sesame oil massage then a shower.

Note: It is important to keep your brush clean. Wash it often with warm soapy water, then allow it to air dry. Once per week treat your brush to a 30-minute soak in a solution of one quart of water and a few drops of Clorox bleach.

Rejuvenating Summer Mini-Indulgences

Going barefoot on your lawn or on the beach for at least 15 minutes a day can help your body get grounded. We are surrounded by invisible electromagnetic pollution day in and day out: microwave ovens, cordless phones, computers, cell phone towers, high-tension wires, and airplanes. When you are grounded, you discharge chaotic electromagnetic energies and absorb healing electrons from the earth through the body. These healing electrons can stop aging and disease by quelling free radicals.

Aromatherapy Baths (20 minutes, 3 times a week before bed)

In summer, soak up the power of aromatherapy baths with lymph-friendly essential oils that also restore cardiovascular harmony and ease digestion:

- Juniper—promotes the elimination of toxic waste and reduces fluid retention
- Lemongrass—tones and strengthens connective tissues and stimulates lymphatic drainage; purges excess fluid from your system
- Grapefruit—antimicrobial; helps dissolve fatty deposits; tones and tightens
- Rose—tones the heart, reduces palpitations, helps circulation
- Fennel—staves off cramps and relieves constipation due to anethole, which is an aromatic component with antispasmodic effects
- Peppermint—alleviates flatulence, bloating, and upset stomach
- Chamomile—calming, quieting, and soothing

16 SUMMER FITNESS PLAN

My favorite part of it all was that I stopped stressing my body out through long, intense workouts...I started enjoying walking, bouncing, and sleeping!

—Emily Jean S., Joliet, Illinois

THE FIRST TWO TO FOUR WEEKS of Summer Fat Flush, you will be in the extreme detox phase of the plan, but "extreme" applies to the diet only, not exercise. The Summer Fitness Plan starts with a gentle exercise program. I know that this may be difficult for you, as you may feel like you should be adding to the intensity of your workouts. But it is essential *not* to incorporate intense exercise during this 14-day period. And this goes if you are extending the extreme Fat Flush diet for up to one month. You are simply not getting the longer-lasting carbohydrates that are required to sustain more vigorous activity. Even if you feel the urge to skip ahead to the next stage, please don't. It is perfectly fine to lighten your exercise load temporarily. Keep in mind that you may be losing up to a pound a day. It is not uncommon to get sluggish during this phase, especially if you are cutting out such quick-fix stimulants as refined carbs, caffeine, and sugar for the first time.

After your time on the extreme detox is over and you've reintroduced some energy-giving Clean Carbs to your diet, you can ease back into more intense workouts. Summer is a great time to get outside, get your lymph flowing, and fill your lungs with fresh air. Swimming, waterskiing, rowing, hiking, and fast-paced walking will get your heart pumping and ensure cardiovascular health. Be sure to get moving at least three days a week for 30 minutes each day.

In the warm weather of summer, it is important to drink enough water to maintain sufficient hydration and avoid such dangers as heat stroke and dehydration. In the summer heat we perspire more, so the risk for dehydration is so much greater. During the hotter months, I want you to avoid antiperspirants like the plague because they hinder the body's natural ability to sweat, which is really nature's own built-in cooling system. This is especially important for women who might be encountering hot flashes and night sweats. Remember, you shed a lot of unwanted toxins out of the body through sweating.

Summer Workout Summary
  (Month 1 during extreme detox)
  Yoga-Quickies *(5 to 10 minutes, 5 days a week) Turn to page 49 in the Pre–Fat Flush Fitness Plan for a description of these moves.*
  Yoga-Quickie Belly Breathing
  Yoga-Quickie Calming Breath
  Yoga-Quickie Poses (1 to 5)

> Please remember to warm up properly before you begin each workout, and cool down with stretching at the end, to lessen soreness and increase flexibility.

  Summer Detox Cardio Workout *(15 minutes, 5 days a week)*
  Workout 1—Ultralight Walkout for Treadmill
  Workout 2—Ultralight Rebounding Routine

  (Months 2 and 3 after extreme detox is complete)
  Yoga-Quickies *(5 to 10 minutes, 5 days a week)*
  Summer Cardio Workout *(35 minutes, 5 days a week)*
  Workout 1—Walkout for Treadmill
  Workout 2—A Walk in the Park
  Workout 3—Rebounding
  Summer Core Exercises *(5 to 10 minutes, 3 nonconsecutive days a week)*

SUMMER DETOX CARDIO WORKOUTS (MONTH 1)

Remember to take it easy during extreme detox and stop exercising if you feel dizzy or otherwise unwell. You'll need to set aside 15 minutes for these exercises (including warm-ups and cool-downs). Be sure to follow the RPE chart on page 57 as directed for each exercise.

Cardio Workout 1: Ultralight Walkout for the Treadmill

Warm-Up Walk 3 minutes; RPE 3–4
Walk   3 minutes, increase speed to 3.5 mph; RPE 5–6
Walk   3 minutes, increase speed to 3.8 mph; RPE 6–7
Walk   3 minutes, decrease speed to 3 mph; increase incline to 4 (pump your arms as you climb); RPE 6–7
Cool-Down Walk 3 minutes; RPE 3–4
Total Workout Time: 15 minutes, including warm-up and cool-down.

> **YOU KNOW YOU ARE A FAT FLUSHER WHEN...** the jeans you couldn't breathe in last week zip up easily today, even though the scale says you're up half a pound.

Cardio Workout 2: Ultralight Rebounding Routine

Warm-Up—3 minutes

Walking slowly in place, raising your legs as high as you can

Cardio Phase—9 minutes

    Light Bounce—3 minutes

  A gentle bounce with feet together or apart

  Jumping Jack Bounce—3 minutes

  A gentle bounce bringing feet together and
apart and raising arms together and apart in
a jumping jack motion

    Heel-Jack Bounce—3 minutes

  A bounce starting with feet together, then
flex the foot and take one heel out, tap the
rebounder and then bring the foot back.
Then, repeat move with opposite foot.

Cool-Down—3 minutes

Walking slowly in place, raising your legs as
  high as you can

*Total Workout Time: 15 minutes, including warm-
up and cool-down*

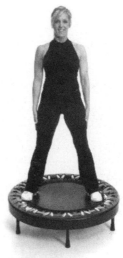

Basic Bounce

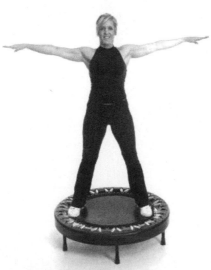

Jumping Jack Bounce

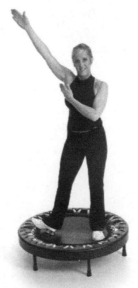

Heel Jack Bounce

Walkout for the Treadmill Routine

Warm-Up Walk	5 minutes; RPE 3–4
Walk	3 minutes, increase speed to 3.5 mph; RPE 5–6
Walk	3 minutes, increase speed to 3.8 mph; RPE 6–7
Walk	5 minutes, decrease speed to 3 mph; increase incline to 5 (pump your arms as you climb); RPE 7–8
Walk	3 minutes, increase speed to 3.5 mph; decrease incline to 0; RPE 3–4
Walk	5 minutes; decrease speed to 2.6 mph; increase incline to 10 (pump your arms as you climb); RPE 8–9
Walk	3 minutes; increase speed to 3.5 mph; decrease incline to 0; RPE 5–6
Walk	3 minutes; increase speed to 3.8 mph; RPE 6–7
Cool-Down Walk	5 minutes; RPE 3–4

Total Workout Time: 35 minutes, including warm-up and cool-down.

SUMMER CARDIO WORKOUTS (MONTHS 2 AND 3)

Now that the accelerated detox portion of summer is over, you can increase your cardio duration and add back core exercises and resistance training.

Cardio Option 1—Walkout for the Treadmill

Duration: 35 minutes; follow Rate of Perceived Exertion (RPE) scale
Frequency: 5 days a week total cardio options
Targets: Cardiovascular and lymphatic systems
Body-Shaping Tools: Walking shoes

Cardio Option 2—A Walk in the Park Interval Training

Duration: 35 minutes; follow instructions for each segment as indicated
Frequency: 5 days a week
Targets: Cardiovascular and lymphatic systems and full body toning
Body-Shaping Tools: Walking shoes

This routine combines cardio interval training with toning. It is an outdoor workout that will blast you into shape and you won't even have to step foot in the gym, though you can do it on a treadmill on very hot summer days.
Turn to page 93 in Winter Fat Flush for a description of these moves.

Warm-Up Segment—Walking
Duration: 5 minutes; RPE 1–3

Cardio Toning Segment 1—Alternating Lunges
Duration: 1 minute; RPE 5–6

Cardio Segment 1—Walking
Duration: 5 minutes; RPE 3–4

Cardio Toning Segment 2—Park Bench Push-ups
Duration: 1 minute; 12 to 15 repetitions; RPE 5–6

Cardio Segment 2—Walking
Duration: 5 minutes; RPE 4–5

Cardio Toning Segment 3—Side Lunges
Duration: 1 minute; 12 to 15 repetitions; RPE 5–6

Cardio Segment 3—Speed Walk or Run
Duration: 5 minutes; RPE 6–7

Cardio Toning Segment 4—Park Bench Dips
Duration: 1 minute; 12–15 repetitions; RPE 5–6
Body-Shaping Tool: Bench

Cardio Segment 4—Speed Walk or Run
Duration: 5 minutes; RPE 6–7

Cardio Toning Segment 5—Skipping
Duration: 1 minute; RPE 5–6

Cool-Down Segment
Duration: 5 minutes; RPE 1–3
Total Workout Time: 35 minutes, includes warm-up and cool-down

Cardio Option 3—Rebounding
Duration: 35 minutes (to the beat of your favorite iPod tunes)
Frequency: 5 days a week

Targets: Cardiovascular and lymphatic systems
Body-Shaping Tools: Rebounder

MODERATE REBOUNDING ROUTINE
Warm-Up Light Bounce—5 minutes
Cardio Phase—25 minutes
    Moderate Bounce—5 minutes
    Moderate Bounce or Jog with Chest Press—2 minutes
    Moderate Bounce or Jog with Shoulder Press—2 minutes
    Moderate Jog—5 minutes
    Moderate Bounce or Jog with Combined Chest and Shoulder Press—2 minutes
    Heel-Jack Bounce—5 minutes
    Jumping Jack Bounce—4 minutes
Cool-Down Light Bounce—5 minutes
Total Workout Time: 35 minutes, including warm-up and cool-down

Turn to page 126 in Spring Fat Flush for a description of these moves.

CORE EXERCISES

Medicine Ball Crunch
Duration: 1 set of 10
Frequency: 3 nonconsecutive days per week

Torso Twist
Duration: 1 set of 10; do set 3 times
Frequency: 3 nonconsecutive days per week

Side Plank
Duration: 1 set of 10; do set 3 times
Frequency: 3 nonconsecutive days per week

Back Extension
Duration: 1 set of 10; do set 3 times
Frequency: 3 nonconsecutive days per week

Turn to page 97 in the Winter Fitness Plan for a full description of these moves.

Part 6
Autumn Fat Flush

17 AUTUMN FAT FLUSH DIET

To eat is a necessity, but to eat intelligently is an art.

—La Rochefoucauld

AS THE AUTUMN LEAVES CHANGE, your body is starting to ready itself for the cold and dark winter months ahead. This is the time to wean off of summer's raw, cooling foods and savor more warming, cooked foods in the forms of soups, stews, and casseroles. With the plummeting temperatures and cold setting in, you need to take special care of the two vital organs of the season: the lungs and the large intestine, both equally important detox organs. Common seasonal symptoms relating to the lungs and large intestine include:

- Sinus headaches, rhinitis, or dry mucous membranes
- Respiratory disorders such as asthma or bronchitis
- Dry cough
- Colitis or diverticulitis
- Foul-smelling stools
- Systemic yeast infections, aches, and pains in joints

To nourish these organs and detox your body from the heavier proteins you've been consuming to this point, you will spend the next three months reaping rewards from the warming spices, legumes, and root vegetables of the vegetarian Fat Flush diet.

Unquestionably, there are well-documented environmental and health advantages to following vegetarian and vegan diets. You know you are doing something good and greener for the planet. Many animal proteins such as beef, poultry, and fish are contaminated with hormones, antibiotics, or mercury. I mean, have you ever heard of mad bean disease? By cutting out animal proteins, you may have a lower risk of heart disease, reduced blood pressure, decreased cancer risk, lower incidences of osteoporosis, and a decreased risk of prostate cancer. Over 12 million vegetarians couldn't be wrong. Besides, economically and for those "flexitarians" out there, vegetarianism makes plain good sense.

PLANT PROTEINS RESET THE METABOLISM

Since the release of *The Fat Flush Plan*, I have become aware of the increasing need for a vegetarian version of the plan. Nowadays, even die-hard carnivores are opting for more veggies, because of their health…and their pocketbooks. That said, my vegetarian Fat Flush addresses weight loss *and* supports optimal physical and emotional health. It provides ample amounts of plant-based protein, which studies have shown allow people to lose more weight than those who consume meat.

In fact, clinical studies have demonstrated plant-based protein is a fat fighter, as it can curb your appetite, supports the weight-loss functions of the liver and the thyroid, and boosts metabolism. A recent study published in the *New England Journal of Medicine* reported that low-carb dieters lost 50 percent more weight by getting most of their protein from plants, compared to those who ate more meat.[1] A look at related research published in the journal *Nutrition Reviews* brought to light that women who on a daily basis ate mostly plant-based protein weighed an average of 15 percent less pounds than did women who ate meat.[2]

Even more supporting research comes out of the University of California–Davis, where a study found a 40 percent reduction in consumed calories for people who ate more plant-based protein. Add to this the fact that plant-based foods are naturally alkaline, helping to offset the acidic diet of carbonated drinks, processed foods, and yes, meats. The plant-based protein helps normalize the body's pH level and allow for more optimum functioning of the liver and the thyroid.

My vegetarian Fat Flush is designed to serve two important purposes: It provides you with a program to detox the body while providing vital nutrition, and prepares your body for the cold weather to come. You will also find *Fat Flush on the Fly* recommendations specifically tailored to your vegetarian needs. This will help you make Fat Flush–friendly food choices when you're time crunched and convenience food becomes necessary.

Teas and Herbs that Cleanse, Heal, and Relax

Fenugreek tea is the premiere fall herbal tea of choice. If you resonate with any of the symptoms that relate to the lungs and colon, I suggest you use one to two cups of Fenugreek tea in addition to the other Fat Flushing beverages. This tea softens and helps to eliminate mucus in the lungs and lubricates the GI tract to prevent constipation.

Specific lung-protecting herbs include usnea, which the Native Americans called "the Lungs of the Earth," because it destroys such pathogenic bacteria as staph, strep, and mycobacterium; osha, a powerful aid for bronchial irritations with immune stimulating properties; mullein, a strong expectorant; and lobelia, a major bronchial dilator and antispasmodic good for lung congestion and asthma. Colon-protecting herbs, such as butternut root bark, function as one of the safest and most effective natural laxatives and parasite removers.

THE UMAMI FACTOR—THE FIFTH TASTE

One feature you will find unique to Autumn's vegetarian Fat Flush is the purposeful use of the umami factor—the "fifth taste." The umami factor adds a kind of meaty, full-bodied flavor and satiety. Many people who have trouble sticking with a meatless diet feel deprived and miss the savoriness and satisfaction of meat. That's why my vegetarian Fat Flush meal plans include such foods as beans (pinto, black, and garbanzo [chickpeas]) and mushrooms (cremini, shiitake, and portobello) in recipes, to provide the mouth feel and fullness of animal proteins. Mushrooms in particular can eliminate hunger pains because they contain nearly 40 percent satiating protein.

For those of you who are looking for flexibility in food choices, take advantage of the Autumn Fat Flushing Superstar Foods, so you can make personalized substitutions wherever your taste buds desire in the menu plans.

THINK ZINC

There is a profound need for vegetarians to keep an eye on their zinc levels. One of the most common deficits (besides that of the well-documented B_{12}) is a lack of zinc, a mineral crucial for proper immunity and reproductive health. Besides being present in pumpkin seeds, the highest amount of zinc is found in red meats, poultry, and seafood (sorry). Plus, the more traditional vegetarian meals where soy and whole grains are emphasized are relatively high in copper, a mineral that is antagonistic to zinc. Cooked whole grains not only contain copper but also are high in phytic acids, which interfere with the absorption of zinc.

As I mentioned earlier in the book, in my own experience I have found that vegetarians are usually zinc deficient and copper toxic. They also have an inversion of the sodium-to-potassium ratio, a sign of adrenal burnout or adrenal insufficiency. When glandular and mineral balance is thrown off, numerous conditions develop, such as low immunity, skin problems, yeast infections, hair loss, depression, and a loss of mental focus.

WHAT DOES COPPER OVERLOAD MEAN TO YOU?

Too much copper can cause anxiety, irritability, and hyperactivity, to name just a few symptoms. Excess copper overstimulates the brain so you are constantly high-strung, resulting in the inability to sleep. Ultimately, copper overload lowers your thyroid gland function so the scale won't budge. It's also tied to acceleration of the aging process, because excess copper causes the breakdown of body protein, leaving you with baggy, loose skin.

PROTEIN POWER

Especially for the vegan Fat Flushers, I have created a powerhouse protein powder that is dairy-(including whey) and soy-free for the most sensitive individuals. Fat Flush Body Protein is made from rice and pea protein (plus stevia and inulin) so that it has a complete balanced profile of amino acids with a respectable 20 grams of protein per serving, and it is GMO-free. This powder blend has a distinct advantage over other vegan protein powders. It balances the high-lysine yellow pea protein with the low-lysine rice protein. Similarly, the high sulfur–bearing cysteine and methionine contained in the rice protein complements the lower levels of these amino acids in the yellow pea. Plus, it even tastes good.

Without complete protein, the thyroid is not able to ignite the fuel that transforms food into energy. The adrenals become exhausted because a high copper level prevents zinc from being bio-available, which results in decreased potassium levels. Even though most vegetarians eat a lot of high-potassium vegetables in their diet, they are unable to retain potassium in the tissues because of a relative zinc deficiency. A typical vegetarian diet is high in vegetables and nuts (raw or uncooked), which are very low in zinc. I have purposefully designed Autumn's vegetarian Fat Flush to include a zinc supplement while limiting high-copper foods such as nuts, soy, chocolate, and regular tea.

> *I have always had dark circles under my eyes and have noticed in the past few days they have been dramatically reduced. I'm on the vegetarian version of the Fat Flush protocol.*
>
> *—Fat Flush fan*

AUTUMN FAT FLUSHING SUPERSTAR FOODS: MONTH 1

In all three months of Autumn, you will enjoy vegetarian-style Fat Flushing Superstar Foods, including ½ cup of beans and one serving of dairy, to make sure your protein needs are met. (Although legumes are technically carbohydrates, they are extremely high in protein.) In addition, the following foods and beverages will help to flush excess fat and toxin-laden fluids from the system: detoxifying beverages, slimming oils, flavorful herbs and spices, fill-you-up veggies and fruits, and even a few "legal cheats." In the succeeding months of Autumn Fat Flush, your food choices will be deliciously expanded upon in the finest culinary Fat Flushing fashion. As with the previous seasonal Fat

> **YOU KNOW YOU ARE A FAT FLUSHER WHEN…** you are wearing pants you wouldn't wear two weeks ago in public!

Flushes, each of the food equivalents are interchangeable with all the others listed in the same group.

Cranberry H₂O

Recipe: See page 198.
Bodily Consumption: 64 ounces per day between each meal and snack, in Green Life Cocktail, and in frappés.

Hot Lemon Water

Recipe: See page 200.
Bodily Consumption: Daily on arising

Green Life Cocktail

Recipe: See page 199.
Bodily Consumption: Daily on arising

Probiotic Sweetener

Benefits: Contains beneficial bacteria to balance GI tract for weight-loss insurance and enhanced immunity. Provides yeast-free sweetener for no-heat frappés, beverages, and desserts.
Brand: UNI KEY's Flora-Key
Bodily Consumption: 1 to 3 teaspoons per day in Green Life Cocktails and frappés and with nonheated foods

Pea and Brown Rice Protein Powder

Benefits: A complete, hypoallergenic, plant-based protein source from peas and brown rice that has a protein efficiency ratio equal to eggs and dairy; assists with lean muscle mass development, increases energy, natural appetite suppressant; dairy- and soy-free for sensitive individuals
Brand: Fat Flush Body Protein
Bodily Consumption: Up to 2 servings per day (20 grams protein each) in frappés, muffins, and desserts

Chia Seeds

Bodily Consumption: 2 to 3 tablespoons per day, added to frappés, soups, stews, and dressings or sprinkled on such foods as eggs and veggies

Slimming Oils

High-lignan Flaxseed Oil
Benefits: Natural anti-inflammatory that inhibits weight gain; helps keep blood sugar levels even, provides satiety and balanced hormones. A good source for omega-3 fatty acids.
Brands: Omega Nutrition, Health from the Sun, and Spectrum

Bodily Consumption: Total of 2 tablespoons per day of flaxseed oil. Do not heat flaxseed oil.

Extra-Virgin Olive Oil in an oil mister (such as Misto)
Bodily Consumption: Lightly spritz in cooking as needed

Herbs, Spices, and Seasonings
Choose from:
Anise
Apple cider vinegar
Bay leaves
Cayenne
Chives (fresh or dried)
Cinnamon
Cloves
Cilantro
Coriander
Cream of tartar
Cumin

Dill (fresh or dried)
Dried mustard
Fennel (fresh or dried)
Garlic (fresh or garlic powder)
Ginger (fresh or dried)
Onion powder
Parsley (fresh or dried)
Turmeric
Wasabi
Bodily Consumption: ¼ to ½ teaspoon at least 3 to 5 times per week

Protein (in addition to 1 to 2 servings daily of Fat Flush Body Protein)
If going meatless isn't your thing, then substitute two four-ounce servings of lean beef, veal, lamb, poultry, fish, or shellfish for the legumes and dairy protein selections below.
To ensure the proper amount of protein, include the following daily:
½ cup legumes
1 serving dairy
Up to 2 omega-enriched eggs (hormone-free/free-range encouraged)
Also include 4 ounces tofu and/or tempeh 2 times per week.

Choose from:
Legumes (cooked)
½ cup red or green lentils
½ cup black, pinto or garbanzo beans

½ cup yellow or green split peas
Brands (canned): Eden with kombu, Westbrae

Dairy

Cheese (hard and semisoft)
Choose from:
  Cheddar
  Feta
  Goat
  Mozzarella
  Parmesan
  Romano
  String
  Swiss
  Bodily Consumption: 1 ounce

Cottage and Ricotta Cheese
Bodily Consumption: ½ cup

Yogurt (plain nonfat, low-fat, or whole milk)
Bodily Consumption: 1 cup

Kefir (plain)
Bodily Consumption: 1 cup

Omega-Enriched Eggs
Bodily Consumption: Up to 2 per day

Other Vegetarian Protein Sources

Choose from:
  Tofu—unflavored, firm and silken (Mori-Nu, White Wave)
  Tempeh (Turtle Island Foods, Lightlife)
  Bodily Consumption: Up to 2 servings (4 ounces each) of tofu and/or tempeh per week

Fruits

Benefits: These low-glycemic fruits are high in vitamin C, natural enzymes, and muscle-sparing potassium and are the best natural snacks on the planet. Look for fresh (without mold) or frozen.

Brands (frozen): Cascadian Farm (www.cfarm.com) or Stahlbush Farms (www.stahlbush.com)

Bodily Consumption: Up to 2 servings per day

Choose from:
  1 small apple, orange, nectarine, peach, pear, or pomegranate
  1 cup berries (blueberries, blackberries, raspberries, and/or cranberries)

6 large strawberries
10 large cherries
2 medium-size plums
½ grapefruit
Lemons and limes (as desired)

Vegetables

Fresh: Look for fresh (in season locally is best) vegetables that are full of vibrant color so that you can eat the rainbow.

Frozen (brands): Frozen vegetables are acceptable as well, such as Woodstock Farms (www.woodstock-farms.com), Cascadian Farm (www.cfarm.com), and Stahlbush Farm (www.stahlbush.com).

Canned: No added salt or sugar

Bodily Consumption: Aim for at least 5 or more servings per day. A vegetable serving is generally 1 cup raw or ½ cup cooked.

Choose from:

(*All unlimited except where noted*)

Artichokes (1 whole or 5 hearts)
Arugula
Asparagus
Bamboo shoots
Bell peppers (red, green, and orange)
Bok choy
Broccoli
Brussels sprouts
Burdock
Cabbage
Carrots (limit 1 medium-size or 5 baby)
Cauliflower
Celery
Celery root
Chard
Chinese cabbage
Chives
Cilantro
Collard greens
Cucumbers
Daikon

Dandelion greens
Eggplant
Endive
Escarole
Green beans
Hearts of palm
Jalapeños
Jerusalem artichoke
Jicama
Kale
Kohlrabi
Leeks
Lettuce (red or green, romaine, butter, baby greens, etc.)
Mushrooms
Mustard greens
Okra
Olives (black, 3 per day)
Onions
Radicchio
Radishes
Rhubarb (1 cup)
Shallots
Snow peas

Spaghetti squash
Spinach
Sprouts (alfalfa, mung bean, broccoli)
Sugar snap peas
Tomatillos
Tomatoes and tomato products (see below)
Water chestnuts
Watercress
Yellow squash
Zucchini

Tomato Products (no added sugar or salt)
Diced tomatoes
Tomato sauce
Pizza sauce
Tomato paste
Tomato puree
Whole peeled tomatoes

Brands: Muir Glen, Eden, Bio Nature, Woodstock Farms

Sea Vegetables

Benefits: Rich in iodine and many trace minerals such as calcium and iron, sea veggies support thyroid function and also inhibit the absorption of radiation and heavy metals.

Choose from: Agar, arame, hijiki, kombu, nori, sea palm fronds, wakame

Brand: Eden

Bodily Consumption: Up to 2 servings of 1 tablespoon agar and/or ½ cup of arame, hijiki, kombu, nori, sea palm fronds, and wakame per week added to soups, stews, poultry, beef, fish, seafood, salads, veggies, eggs, etc.

You may also add a sea veggie–based seasoning:

Brand: Eden Seaweed Gomasio (contains sea vegetables, sesame seeds, and sea salt)

Bodily Consumption: ½ teaspoon daily

Beverages

Healing Tea
Fenugreek tea

Brands: Alvita and Traditional Medicinals

Bodily Consumption: 1 to 2 cups per day

Legal Cheats (optional)

Organic coffee (caffeinated)
Bodily Consumption: 1 cup each day

Salt
Bodily Consumption: ½ to 1 teaspoon per day. (Use your best judgment— if you bloat, are hypertensive, or take a diuretic, then take less. If you have low blood pressure or suffer from adrenal exhaustion, you can use up to 1 teaspoon per day.)

Stevia Plus (for use in heated foods)
Bodily Consumption: Maximum of 2 packets per day

AUTUMN FAT FLUSHING SUPERSTARS: MONTH 2

Here you will find even more healthy eating choices that will make menu planning for Month 2 more varied. I have included brand-new superfoods that you can enjoy in addition to the Month 1 staples, including some Clean Carbs. They provide a treasure chest of phytonutrients such as carotenoids (sweet potatoes), fiber (bread and tortillas), and cancer-fighting isothiocyanates (rutabagas and turnips) that will enable you to eat better and feel better while continuing to lose weight. I've even added some alcohol—in moderation, of course—to lift your spirits.

Use these in addition *to your Autumn Fat Flushing Superstar Foods: Month 1 (page 166):*

Spiced Lemon Toddy
Recipe: See page 200.
Bodily Consumption: Daily on arising

Herbs, Spices, and Seasonings
Choose from: (fresh or dried)

Basil (fresh or dried)

Chinese five-spice powder

Dijon mustard (without added sugar)

Mint (fresh or dried)

Oregano (fresh or dried)

Rosemary (fresh or dried)

Bodily Consumption: ¼ to ½ teaspoon at least 3 to 5 times per week

CLEAN CARBS

Once again, start with small bites to make sure you don't bloat, have gas, or develop headaches. In the first two weeks, try one serving each day of a starchy veggie carb (such as 1 small sweet potato or yam) and see how you do. If all goes well, in the remaining two weeks, try two Clean Carb servings (total) each day, which can now include selections from the Bread and Tortilla and Grains and Cereal groups.

Choose from:

1 small sweet potato or yam

½ cup green peas

½ cup carrots

½ cup winter squash (such as butternut, Delicata, hubbard, acorn, and kabocha)

½ cup parsnips

½ cup pumpkin (fresh and unsweetened pure canned)

½ cup turnips

½ cup rutabagas

Bread and Tortillas
Choose from: French Meadow Healthseed Spelt Bread (yeast-free); Kinnikinnick Candadi Multigrain Rice Bread (yeast- and gluten-free); and Food for Life Ezekiel 4:9 Sprouted Whole Grain Tortilla (yeast- and gluten-free)
Bodily Consumption: 1 slice bread or 1 (6-inch) tortilla

Grains and Cereals

Quinoa
Bodily Consumption: ½ cup cooked

Oatmeal (rolled, quick, or steel-cut)
Bodily Consumption: ½ cup cooked

Legal Cheats

Alcohol (grain-free)
Choose from:
    Potato vodka
    Rum (made from sugar)
    Tequila (from the cactus plant)
Bodily Consumption: 1 ounce mixed
with water, Cranberry H_2O, or unflavored sparkling water once a week

Sparkling water (unflavored)
Bodily Consumption: 8 ounces, 2 to 3 times per week

AUTUMN FAT FLUSHING SUPERSTAR FOODS: MONTH 3

Following, you will find more sustaining and substantial nutritional options to integrate into late autumn. Use these additional Fat Flush Superstar Foods to widen your variety of healthy food choices for lifelong weight control, long-term satiety, and well-being.

Use these along with your Month 1 (page 166) and Month 2 Autumn Fat Flushing Superstar Foods (page 170):

Slimming Oils

Choose 1 tablespoon from the following oils in addition to *the tablespoon of flaxseed oil:*
    Extra-virgin olive oil
    Macadamia nut oil
    Coconut oil
    Sesame oil

Herbs, Spices, and Seasonings

Choose from:
    Allspice
    Caraway seeds (1 teaspoon)
    Cardamom
    Horseradish
    Marjoram (fresh or dried)
    Nutmeg
    Poppy seeds (1 teaspoon)
    Saffron
    Sage (fresh or dried)
    Savory (fresh or dried)
    Tarragon (fresh or dried)
    Thyme (fresh or dried)
Bodily Consumption: ¼ to ½ teaspoon at least 3 to 5 times per week

Clean Carbs

In Month 3, add a third Clean Carb to your daily intake and choose from the seasonal selections below. You can even add a second serving of dairy and legumes, if you choose.

Starchy Vegetables
Choose from:
- ½ cup beets (red or golden)
- ½ cup corn, or 1 ear corn on the cob
- ½ cup potatoes, or 1 small baked
- ½ cup whole-grain pasta (Hodgson Mill)
- ½ cup spelt or rice pasta (Tinkyada, Eden)
- ½ cup toasted buckwheat or amaranth cereal
- 3 cups plain popcorn (popped)

Tortillas, Crackers, and Chips
Choose from:
- 1 corn tortilla (Food for Life)
- 2 Scandinavian-style crispbreads (Wasa, Kauli, Bran-a-Crisp)
- 5 brown rice crackers
- 7 blue corn chips

Cereals and Grains (cooked)
Choose from:
- ½ cup brown or wild rice (Lundberg Family Farms)

Legumes (when cooked acts as both a Clean Carb and Protein)
Choose from:
- ½ cup red or green lentils
- ½ cup black, pinto, or garbanzo beans (chickpeas)
- ½ cup yellow or green split peas

Dairy
Cheese (hard and semisoft)

Choose from:

- Cheddar
- Feta
- Goat
- Mozzarella
- Parmesan
- Romano
- String
- Swiss

Bodily Consumption: 1 ounce

Cottage and Ricotta Cheese
Bodily Consumption: ½ cup

Yogurt (plain nonfat, low-fat, or whole milk)
Bodily Consumption: 1 cup

Kefir (plain)
Bodily Consumption: 1 cup

Nuts, Seeds, Nut Butters, and Friendly Fats

7 almonds or filberts

3 macadamia nuts

4 pecan or walnut halves

4 large chestnuts

1 tablespoon seeds (sesame, pumpkin, and/or sunflower)

1 tablespoon almond, peanut, and/or sesame-tahini butter (Westbrae, Arrowhead Mills, Marantha)

½ small avocado

1 tablespoon cream cheese

1 tablespoon sour cream

1 pat of butter

1 tablespoon unsweetened coconut

Bodily Consumption: 1 serving per day

Beverages (optional)

Vegetable Juices

Benefits: High in antioxidants and vitamins; adds variety to beverage choices

Brands: V8 Juice, Knudsen Organic Very Veggie Juice

Bodily Consumption: 8 ounces per day

Legal Cheats (optional)

Cocoa Powder

Bodily Consumption: 1 teaspoon, once a week

Carob Powder

Bodily Consumption: 1 teaspoon, once a week

Cacao Powder

Bodily Consumption: 1 teaspoon, once a week

Flavor Extracts

Choose from:

Almond

Anise

Lemon

Mint

Orange

Rum

Vanilla

Bodily Consumption: ¼ to ½ teaspoon, as needed

A GENTLE REMINDER—ESPECIALLY FOR AUTUMN FAT FLUSH

- Menu plans are completely optional. If following a structured plan is not for you, feel free to create your own fabulous Fat Flush-friendly meals and snacks that follow the guidelines for Autumn.
- Recipes noted with an asterisk (*) appear in chapter 21.
- Lunches, dinners, and snacks are interchangeable within the same day.
- You may add an extra tablespoon of chia seeds into recipes, if desired.
- Make sure to drink a total of 64 ounces of Cranberry H_2O daily between meals. Eight ounces are included in a daily Green Life Cocktail. You may also drink plain filtered water (as much as you'd like), provided you have consumed the recommended 64 ounces of Cranberry H_2O. In addition, 1 daily cup of organic coffee and/or 1 to 2 cups of fenugreek tea is also acceptable.
- Continue to optimize your results with the Fat Flush Kit supplements: the Dieters' Multi (with or without iron) for balanced vitamin and mineral supplementation; the GLA 90s for stimulating brown adipose tissue metabolism which increases fat burning and keeps skin moist and taut during weight loss; and the Weight Loss Formula for carbohydrate control, fat metabolism, and liver support (without stimulants). Also continue to take 1,000 mg of CLA three times per day with meals.
- Take a zinc supplement of 50 to 100 mg daily.

AUTUMN FAT FLUSH: 14-DAY MEAL PLANNER (MONTH 1)
DAY 1

On Arising
Hot Lemon Water* (page 200)
Green Life Cocktail* (page 199)

Breakfast
Berry Wonderful Frappé* (page 201)

Snack
½ cup plain hummus
Endive leaves and orange pepper sticks

Fat Flush on the Fly: Tribe Hummus

Lunch
Sunshine Frittata* (page 206) with 1 tablespoon of chia seeds
1 nectarine

Snack
1 ounce cheddar cheese
Snow peas and cauliflower florets

Dinner
2 cups veggie broth with green onion,
snow peas, and 4 ounces of tofu
Baby greens and watercress salad with 1
tablespoon each of flaxseed oil and
freshly squeezed lemon juice

DAY 2

On Arising
Hot Lemon Water* (page 200)
Green Life Cocktail* (page 199)

Breakfast
Berries 'n' Cherries Frappé* (page 202)

Snack
2 cups Just Vegg'n-Out Munchies* (page 248)

Lunch
½ cup cottage cheese with 1 teaspoon of Flora-Key and ground cinnamon
Baby spinach salad with grated daikon radish, carrot, and freshly squeezed lime juice

Snack
1 Fabulous Chia Crax* (page 246) sprinkled with 1 teaspoon of Flora-Key
1 orange

Dinner
2 cups Ethiopian Lentil Stew* (page 222) mixed with 1 tablespoon of chia seeds
Steamed kale with garlic and freshly squeezed lemon juice

Timesaver Tip! *Save leftover stew for Day 4's Lunch.*

DAY 3

On Arising
Hot Lemon Water* (page 200)
Green Life Cocktail* (page 199)

Breakfast
Artichoke Omelet made with 2 eggs, 3 chopped artichoke hearts, chopped parsley, and ground cumin

Snack
Blueberry Vanilla Frappé* (page 202)

Lunch
Dragon Bowl Salad* (page 219) made with 1 ounce goat cheese and 2 tablespoons E-Z Fat Flush Vinaigrette* (page 237)

Snack
Raspberry Truffle Frappé* (page 202), omitting the flaxseed oil and chia seeds

Dinner
1 Black Bean Cake* (page 223) with salsa
Steamed baby bok choy with garlic

Fat Flush on the Fly: *No time to make homemade salsa? Look for brands without added sugar, such as Muir Glen and Seeds of Change.*

Timesaver Tip! *Save a leftover Black Bean Cake for Day 5's Lunch.*

DAY 4

On Arising
   Hot Lemon Water* (page 200)
   Green Life Cocktail* (page 199)

Breakfast
   Orange Creamsicle Frappé* (page 202)

Snack
   2 cups Just Vegg'n-Out Munchies* (page 248)

Lunch
   2 cups leftover Ethiopian Lentil Stew*
   Shredded red cabbage and carrots with 1 tablespoon of apple cider vinegar

Snack
   1 Fabulous Chia Crax* (page 246) sprinkled with 1 teaspoon of Flora-Key
   1 pear

Dinner
   Squash Ribbons with Creamy Dill Sauce, made with 1 each zucchini and yellow squash, shredded. Heat ¼ cup each of plain yogurt and ricotta cheese. Stir in ½ ounce of grated Romano cheese, fresh dill, and cayenne. Continue to heat the sauce until the cheese melts; toss with the squash
   Warm asparagus with a pinch of Fat Flush Seasoning* (page 235)

DAY 5

On Arising
   Hot Lemon Water* (page 200)
   Green Life Cocktail* (page 199)

Breakfast
   Blackberry Blast Frappé* (page 201)

Snack
   2 cups Just Vegg'n–Out Munchies* (page 248)

Lunch
   Black Bean Cake* Lettuce Wraps made with 1 leftover Black Bean Cake*, chopped peppers, red onion, and salsa wrapped in large lettuce leaves

Snack
   Apple Pie in a Cup made with 1 cup of plain yogurt mixed with 1 chopped apple, ground cinnamon and ginger, and 1 teaspoon of Flora-Key

Dinner
   2 cups 'Shrooms 'n' Tempeh Chili* (page 222)
   Warm green beans with lemon

DAY 6

On Arising
Hot Lemon Water* (page 200)
Green Life Cocktail* (page 199)

Breakfast
Pears 'n' Cinnamon Frappé* (page 202)

Snack
½ cup Roasted Eggplant Spread* (page 247)
Jicama slices and sugar snap peas

Lunch
Toasted Nori and Swiss Cheese made with
1 sheet of toasted nori topped with 1
ounce of Swiss cheese and a pinch of
Seaweed Gomasio. Bake at 400°F until
the cheese is bubbly.

Escarole and dandelion greens tossed with
1 tablespoon each of flaxseed oil and
freshly squeezed lime juice

Snack
1 Fabulous Chia Crax* (page 246) sprinkled
with 1 teaspoon of Flora-Key

Dinner
Chickpeas and "Spaghetti" made with ½
cup of chickpeas cooked with cremini
mushrooms, seeded and chopped red
and green bell peppers, ground coriander, and cayenne, served over steamed
spaghetti squash

DAY 7

On Arising
Hot Lemon Water* (page 200)
Green Life Cocktail* (page 199)

Breakfast
Choco-Rhuberry Frappé* (page 202)

Snack
½ cup Roasted Eggplant Spread* (page 247)
Celery sticks and 5 baby carrots

Lunch
Pinto Bean and Mozzarella Lettuce Wraps
made with ½ cup of pinto beans
cooked with chopped green onions,
peppers, turmeric, cayenne, and 1
ounce of shredded mozzarella cheese,
wrapped in large lettuce leaves

Snack
1 peach, sliced and sprinkled with ground
ginger and 1 tablespoon of chia seeds

Dinner
2 Egg, Portobello, and Spinach Towers*
(page 206)
Chopped cucumbers and parsley with 1
tablespoon each of flaxseed oil and
freshly squeezed lime juice and a pinch
of Seaweed Gomasio

DAY 8

On Arising
Hot Lemon Water* (page 200)
Green Life Cocktail* (page 199)

Breakfast
Peach Melba Frappé* (page 202)

Snack
½ cup Crunchy Chickpeas* (page 249)
Broccoli and cauliflower florets

Lunch
Shiitake Mushroom and Swiss Omelet
made with 2 eggs, ½ cup of shiitake
mushrooms, 1 ounce of Swiss cheese,
chopped fresh cilantro, and a pinch of
Fat Flush Seasoning* (page 235)

6 large strawberries with 1 teaspoon of
Flora-Key

Snack
½ cup Chunky Artichoke Dip* (page 247)
Sugar snap peas and red bell pepper sticks

Dinner
2 cups Szechuan Tofu with Eggplant*
(page 221)
Steamed baby spinach with a pinch of
Seaweed Gomasio and 1 tablespoon of
chia seeds

DAY 9

On Arising
Hot Lemon Water* (page 200)
Green Life Cocktail* (page 199)

Breakfast
Pears 'n' Cinnamon Frappé* (page 202),
omitting the flaxseed oil

Snack
½ cup Chunky Artichoke Dip* (page 247)
Jicama and zucchini rounds (raw)

Lunch
Dragon Bowl Salad* (page 219) made with
1 ounce of mozzarella cheese and 2
tablespoons of E-Z Fat Flush Vinaigrette* (page 237)

Snack
Choco-Cherry Oblivion Frappé* (page 201),
omitting the flaxseed oil

Dinner
2 cups Dhal* (page 224)
Steamed chard with lemon

Timesaver Tip! *Save leftover Dhal for Day 10's
Lunch.*

DAY 10

On Arising
Hot Lemon Water* (page 200)
Green Life Cocktail* (page 199)

Breakfast
Blueberry Mini Chiacakes* (page 204)

Snack
Broccoli florets and yellow squash rounds
with 2 tablespoons of salsa

Lunch
2 cups leftover Dhal
Steamed eggplant with garlic and 1 tablespoon of flaxseed oil

Snack
Rhubarb-Berry Burst Frappé* (page 202)

Dinner
½ Confetti Veggie and Cheddar Quiche
made with 2 beaten eggs, seeded and
diced red pepper, zucchini, yellow
squash, dill, and 2 ounces of shredded
cheddar cheese. Pour into an 11 × 7-
inch baking dish; bake at 350°F for 25
minutes, or until set
Fennel braised in veggie broth with
cayenne

Timesaver Tip! Save half of the quiche for
Day 11's Lunch.

DAY 11

On Arising
Hot Lemon Water* (page 200)
Green Life Cocktail* (page 199)

Breakfast
Just Cherries Frappé* (page 201)

Snack
Cauliflower florets and sugar snap peas
with ½ cup of Crunchy Chickpeas*
(page 249)

Lunch
leftover Confetti Veggie and Cheddar
Quiche

Warm asparagus with a pinch of Fat Flush
Seasoning* (page 235) and 1 tablespoon of chia seeds

Snack
2 plums

Dinner
2 cups Cucumber, Wakame, and Tofu
Salad* (page 220)

DAY 12

On Arising
  Hot Lemon Water* (page 200)
  Green Life Cocktail* (page 199)

Breakfast
  Orange Creamsicle Frappé* (page 202)

Snack
  Jicama sticks and 5 baby carrots with lime
    juice

Lunch
  Veggie Wraps made with seeded and
    chopped bell pepper, celery, broccoli
    sprouts, and salsa, wrapped in Spinach
    "Flatbread"* (page 245)

Snack
  Peach Pie in a Cup made with 1 cup of
    plain yogurt mixed with 1 chopped
    peach, ground cloves and ginger, and 1
    teaspoon of Flora-Key

Dinner
  2 cups Sautéed Escarole with Chickpeas*
    (page 224)
  Steamed spaghetti squash with a pinch of
    Fat Flush Seasoning* (page 235)
  and 1 tablespoon of flaxseed oil

  Timesaver Tip! *Save leftover escarole and
    chickpeas for Day 13's Lunch.*

DAY 13

On Arising
  Hot Lemon Water* (page 200)
  Green Life Cocktail* (page 199)

Breakfast
  Snappy Egg Salad made with 2 hard-boiled
    eggs, chopped celery, red onion, and
    dry mustard, plus 2 tablespoons of E-Z
    Classic Mayo* (page 235)
  Romaine lettuce dippers

  Fat Flush on the Fly: *No time to make
    homemade mayo? Look for Spectrum's
    Omega-3 Mayonnaise with Flax Oil.*

Snack
  Blackberry Blast Frappé* (page 201)

Lunch
  2 cups leftover Sautéed Escarole with
    Chickpeas mixed with 1 tablespoon of
    chia seeds
  Steamed broccoli with a pinch of Seaweed
    Gomasio

Snack
  1 pear

Dinner
  1 serving Spinach- and Goat Cheese–
    Stuffed Portobellos* (page 225)
  Steamed cauliflower mashed with veggie
    broth and dill

DAY 14

On Arising
Hot Lemon Water* (page 200)
Green Life Cocktail* (page 199)

Breakfast
Berries 'n' Cherries Frappé* (page 202)

Snack
¼ cup Lemony Tapenade* (page 248)
Snow peas and 5 baby carrots

Lunch
Roasted Tomatoes Romano made with
roasted tomatoes spritzed with olive
oil, plus chopped fresh parsley and 1
ounce of grated Romano cheese. Roast
in a 350°F oven for 20 minutes.

Arugula and watercress with diced red
onion and 1 tablespoon of apple cider
vinegar

Snack
1 nectarine

Dinner
1 Black Bean Cake* (page 223) with ¼ cup
of Roasted Red Pepper Sauce* (page
236)
Warm green beans with lime and ground
coriander

18 AUTUMN WELLNESS PROGRAM

AUTUMN IS A GREAT TIME TO FINE-TUNE your supplement program. A tissue mineral analysis (TMA) test will help you to determine a personalized supplement program that is more tailor-made for your unique biochemical needs. It can also help detect if there are any glandular issues involved with your weight-loss efforts. In over two decades of working with tissue analysis, I have found that TMA is a much more a reliable guide to thyroid status than are conventional blood tests. TMA reflects how the thyroid hormone is utilized on the cellular level (via the calcium/potassium ratio) over a three-month period of time, whereas blood values of thyroid (TSH, T3, T4) reflect the circulating amounts just in the bloodstream.

When you send in a sample of hair for analysis, you can obtain levels of your stored copper, zinc, calcium, and other minerals. I often tell my clients to think of a hair analysis test as being similar to the reading of the rings of a cut tree. You can tell a great deal about the climate by examining the variations in the rings.

Healing Autumn Rituals

- Record your foods, supplements, exercise, and special reflections in a journal.
- Set aside one day each week to rest, reflect, and regenerate (Sabbath Ritual).
- Irrigate your nose twice daily, upon arising and before bed. Pollutants such as molds and dust, especially in the autumn, can bombard the nasal passages, inhibiting breathing and irritating sensitive mucus membranes. A daily *gravity-flow, saltwater nasal rinse* can reduce swelling, loosen mucus, keep the tissue healthier, and keep your nasal passages hydrated and free from any pollen or debris. Simply dissolve ½ teaspoon of plain, noniodized salt and baking soda in 8 ounces of filtered, warm water in a neti pot or nasal bulb. Stand in front of the sink, and bending forward with your head tilted keeping your mouth open, apply the pot or bulb snugly against your nasal passage and allow the water to drain from the opposite nasal passage. Repeat on other side. For more severe or chronic sinusitis, you may wish to consider pulsed irrigation. There is an FDA-approved sinus flushing device known as the Grossan Hydro Pulse nasal/sinus irrigation system, available in pharmacies or online.

Your hair contains a blueprint, metabolically speaking, of how your body is functioning on a cellular level. It is a simple, noninvasive method for detecting mineral imbalances and in turn correcting them and improving overall wellness as well as weight-loss success. Because I see so much copper imbalance in my clients, it's particularly helpful for knowing whether you should be eliminating excess copper, a mineral that can often depress thyroid function, creating a metabolic meltdown due to copper overload. (For information on ordering, see resources, page 257.)

AUTUMN BACH FLOWER REMEDY

The Autumn Bach Flower Remedy is Crabapple. Known as "the cleanser flower," it is ideal for autumn cleansing because it is designed for individuals who feel both emotionally and physically toxic and want to do something about it.

> **YOU KNOW YOU ARE A FAT FLUSHER WHEN...** you find yourself going out to eat less and enjoying it more.

I suggest that you add four drops of Crabapple to 8 ounces of plain filtered water four times per day and sip it at intervals throughout the day. Remember, you can also put this on your skin or in your bath in the same amounts.

ADVANCED AUTUMN DETOX TECHNIQUES

Do daily **oil pulling** for 10 to 15 minutes upon arising.

Coffee Enema (30 minutes; once or twice per week throughout autumn)

This enema helps the liver and gall bladder in their continued cleansing processes and also clears out the lower colon. The caffeine from the coffee targets the GI tract's portal vein, which carries it to your liver, resulting in a bile dump from the liver's bile ducts (remember that the bile is your body's toxic waste dump). This keeps your body's most important cleansing organ in tip-top shape, resulting in an enhanced immune system. Coffee both cleanses the pathway (acting as an astringent) and stimulates bile flow (enhancing digestion). This advanced detox technique is particularly helpful to slow-oxidizers who tend to have sluggish activity in their liver and digestive tract. Although I am only recommending the coffee enema once or twice per week, do keep in mind that it can be used more frequently for those with more serious conditions.

To get started you will need four items: water, organic coffee, an enema/douche bag with a clamp, and a natural herbal lubricant such as coconut oil or aloe vera.

1. Boil 1 quart of pure water in a stainless-steel, glass, or enamel container.
2. Pour the water through a coffee filter containing 1 teaspoon to 4 tablespoons of ground organic coffee, depending on your tolerance for caffeine (if you are sensitive to caffeine, do this early in the day to avoid sleep disturbances). Start with weak coffee. Do not boil the coffee. Percolated coffee is okay.
3. Hang the enema bag no higher than 2 feet above the floor (any higher will cause it to flow with too much force).
4. Connect the rectal tubing to the end of the bag and seal off the tube with the clamp.
5. Pour the coffee into the bag, allowing a little to run out of the tube, to ensure that there is no air in the tube and that the coffee is not too hot.
6. Lubricate several inches of the rectal tubing and insert it into rectum while lying on your left side. (Note that the length of tubing varies greatly depending on your body and comfort level, so never force tubing in. It may take several enemas before you are comfortable.)
7. Unclamp the tube to allow for the coffee to flow—adjust the flow as needed for comfort.
8. When the flow is done and all coffee has entered your body, you can either remove the tube or leave it in (make sure you remove the clamp to allow any gas that is released from the colon to escape).
9. Gently massage your abdomen for 5 minutes, while lying on your left side. Then repeat while lying on your back and then on your right side.
10. After 5 minutes in each position (15 minutes) sit on the toilet and expel the coffee. If you feel that you can't wait this long—don't. It's important not to strain while doing this enema.

> ## Rejuvenating Autumn Mini-Indulgences
>
> Take time out of your hectic schedule to allow yourself to slow down and rest. If you can, go to bed early or sleep late, twice a week.
>
> Take in the rich tones of autumn by going for an invigorating hike or bike ride. Or take a scenic drive in the country to enjoy the flamboyancy of the season.

Consider trying **colon hydrotherapy treatments**, which ensure regularity in addition to relieving a number of other symptoms including dark circles and bags under your eyes, fatigue, gas, irritability, and headaches. This method irrigates the entire 5 ½-foot length of the large intestines or colon with filtered lukewarm water. It removes hard-to-reach toxins from bulges and pockets where waste material may have been lodging, enabling them to reform back into their original shape. This detox method should be done by a certified colon hydrotherapist. Many people find that they also get moist, radiant skin from this treatment—a welcome alternative to dry, itchy skin typical in the fall.

Aromatherapy (20 minutes; three times per week)

Soak up the power of **aromatherapy** three times a week for 20 minutes by bathing or breathing in essential oils such as cedarwood, eucalyptus, and myrrh (10 drops in bath, 5 drops in small diffuser, or 1 drop on a tissue that is held in front of your nose for a minute or two):

- Cedarwood—fortifies and strengthens the lungs; promotes improved sleep
- Eucalyptus—relieves sinus pressure due to inflammation or infection and clears histamines
- Myrrh—reduces mucus in the intestinal tract and in the lungs.

19 AUTUMN FITNESS PLAN

AUTUMN HAS ARRIVED, and the workouts will vary in intensity based on each month's eating plan. You will start slowly, as the first month of the Autumn Fat Flush is similar to the extreme detox portion of Summer Fat Flush. Through the following two months, you'll increase the duration of your cardio workouts, add back advanced moves to your rebounding routine, and continue to strengthen and shape your new body with core exercises. Go outside and enjoy the weather as often as possible before winter drives you inside. Natural sunlight is a key to the cyclical depression syndrome known as seasonal affective disorder (SAD), which occurs in the fall when daylight hours start to diminish. Depression and overeating (especially carbohydrates) often begin in the fall when daylight lessens. This is the perfect time to emphasize the Basic Breathing exercises that are incorporated in the Yoga Quickies. These poses will help to release any backed-up waste that may be building up in your colon.

Great autumn exercises include aerobic walking, cycling, jumping rope (or, of course, your rebounding), and martial arts. When you are exercising outside, even if the weather is still warm, protect your neck with a scarf. According to ancient Asians, the back of the neck is most vulnerable to autumn wind chills.

Autumn Cardio Workout Summary
Month 1 (extreme detox phase)
    Yoga-Quickies (*5 to 10 minutes, 5 days a week*) *Turn to page 49 in the Pre–Fat Flush Fitness Plan for a description of these moves.*
    Autumn Detox Cardio Workout (*15 minutes, 5 days a week*)
    Workout 1—Ultralight Walkout for Treadmill
    Workout 2—Ultralight Rebounding Routine

During the first month of Autumn Fat Flush, you'll be following a strict detox plan, so you'll need to shorten the duration and intensity of your workouts. You'll be performing the same cardio workouts featured in the Summer Fitness Plan, so turn to page 153 for a refresher on the exercises.

Month 2
    Yoga-Quickies (*5 to 10 minutes, 5 days a week*)
    Moderate Cardio Workouts (*35 minutes for Workouts 1 and 2; 20 minutes for Workout 3; 5 days a week, select Workout 1, 2, or 3*)

Workout 1—Walkout for Treadmill
Workout 2—A Walk in the Park
Workout 3—Rebounding
Core Exercises (*5 to 10 minutes, 3 nonconsecutive days a week*)

Month 2 transitions you back into longer cardio workouts and core exercises. These are the same workouts for Spring Fitness, so turn to page 124 for a more detailed explanation of the routine.

Month 3

Yoga-Quickies (*5 to 10 minutes, 5 days a week*)
Cardio Workouts (*45 minutes for Workouts 1 and 2; 25 minutes for Workout 3; 5 days a week, select Workout 1, 2, or 3*)
Workout 1—Walkout for the Treadmill
Workout 2—A Walk in the Park Cardio Tone Segment
Workout 3—Rebounding
Core Exercises (*5 to 10 minutes, 3 nonconsecutive days a week*)

In month 3, as your Clean Carb intake increases, so too will the intensity and duration of your workouts. You can alternate between two 45-minute cardio workouts and a 25-minute rebounding workout. This is the same program that is recommended for Winter Fitness, so turn to page 92 for information on any of the exercises.

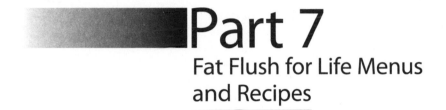

Part 7

Fat Flush for Life Menus and Recipes

20 YEAR-ROUND MENUS FOR FEASTS AND FESTIVITIES

Special occasions can cause even the most organized person to become stressed. Maybe that's why there is a typical ten- to fifteen-pound weight gain between Thanksgiving and New Year's. Dividing our precious time between work, family, and social commitments often leaves us with little time for planning everyday meals...let alone for the holidays.

Here's a real-life scenario: your sister has convinced you that she just can't "do Thanksgiving" this year and begs you to do it. You start to panic. Not only do you normally not cook large family holiday dinners, but you're really worried about creating a delicious but healthy meal that your non–Fat Flushing relatives will savor. Not to worry: a bountiful and flavor-packed Fat Flush for Life crowd-pleasing meal can be enjoyed by all. Whether it be a Thanksgiving Buffet, or Christmas or Hanukkah Spread, Winter Vegetarian Buffet, Romantic Valentine's Dinner for Two, or Fourth of July Barbecue, your menu planning search ends right here!

This chapter is a complete guide to worry-free, Fat Flush–friendly entertaining throughout the year with complete meal plans and recipes. Because celebrations and holidays are the time when trans fats, white sugar, and white flour really take center stage, I have put together an ensemble of Fat Flushing Superstar Foods or recommended "healthy cheats" to be used during just such occasions so that you (or your guests) won't feel deprived. The reality is that you are balancing between "legally cheating" *and* representing the healthiest and highest nutritional value foods for each category. For example, natural sweeteners other than the suggested probiotic sweetener stand up to heat and provide "sweeter" cooked dishes and desserts, while allowing you to avoid the white sugar that is typically used at this time of year.

No matter what season of the year, if you have already reached your goal weight, you will find that you can probably "legally" cheat (in moderation of course) without a blip on the scale. If you have not yet reached your desired weight, just remember that it is what you do every day that counts, not what you eat once in a while—such as on holidays or special events.

But, if you do overeat and overly cheat, especially on sweets and alcohol, which can set off a yeast-feeding frenzy linked to bloating fatigue and food cravings, I have that covered, too—with my Fat Flush Fix (see page 193). If you do overindulge during the holidays, it usually takes three to four days to get back on track.

You will also find that each recipe referenced in the menus in this section has been marked with an asterisk (*). If you are making these recipes for company, make sure that the serving size is appropriately adjusted for the number of guests. For the most part, recipes have been designed to serve four, to accommodate everyday cooking needs. That being said, also keep in mind that not everyone will eat a full portion of every dish. In fact, when a large variety of dishes are offered, many guests typically choose only a few. So relax and enjoy this time with your friends and loved ones!

> *Having started on December 31, today marks one month of successful Fat Flushing. It has been a month of good choices, learning, and rewards. I am well on the way to attaining a more reasonable weight, and the relief to my arthritic knees is already evident—giving hope that putting off replacement surgery is a real possibility. This is cause for a real celebration as anyone with chronic pain issues can understand.*
>
> —Nina, Fat Flush Fan

FAT FLUSHING FESTIVE SUPERSTAR FOODS

Regardless of the season, here follows a list of recommended "healthy cheats" to be used during special times so that you (or your family and guests) won't feel deprived during special gatherings and festive occasions:

YOU KNOW YOU ARE A FAT FLUSHER WHEN... Stevia is too sweet.

Tahini
Benefit: Provides antioxidants such as sesamol
Brand: Arrowhead Mills
Bodily Consumption: Up to 1 tablespoon

The Fat Flush Fix for When You Overeat and Overly Cheat

Celebrations and holidays are notorious for overindulging in foods and drinks. In a short time, all too many of us take in way too much sugar, white flour, and alcohol. Since we are all human, there is no need to beat yourself up if you have overindulged. Just follow the following steps for the Fat Flush Fix. Note that this is absolutely not an excuse to overeat and it will not get rid of the extra pounds you put on—but it will help to cut down on bloating and yeast-related problems.

- Drink plenty of water to help flush your system.
- Up your probiotic to "crowd out" the overgrown yeast in your GI tract.
- Take Y-C Cleanse, a clinically proven homeopathic for the safe and effective treatment of **Candida albicans** and related yeast infections. Y-C works to gently yet effectively treat **Candida** and its friends—available through UNI KEY Health Systems (see resources, page 257).

Aluminum-Free Baking Powder
Benefit: Helps baked products to rise
Brands: Frontier, Rumford, Clabber Girl, Calumet
Bodily Consumption: As needed in baking

Cream
Benefit: Provides healthy saturated fat for strong nerves and satisfied taste buds
Choose: Heavy cream, whipped cream
Bodily Consumption: 2 tablespoons of heavy cream, 4 tablespoons of whipped cream

Almond Milk
Benefits: Provides a dairy alternative for vegans and sensitive individuals; good source of calcium, and vitamins A, D, and E
Choose: Plain unsweetened almond milk
Brand: Blue Diamond
Bodily Consumption: 1 cup

Coconut Milk (unsweetened)
Benefits: Rich in potassium and heart-healthy fat; antiviral and antimicrobial
Brands: Thai Kitchen, Eden
Bodily Consumption: 1 cup

Fruits, Juices, and Sweeteners

The following foods may be used in place of one or more Winter Fat Flush or Autumn Fat Flush Month 3 fruits.

Fruits

Benefit: Natural sweeteners high in enzyme power

Choose: ½ small mango, ⅓ papaya, or ½ cup of unsweetened applesauce

Dried Fruits (unsulfured)

Benefits: Natural sweeteners high in minerals such as iron, potassium, and calcium

Choose from: 1 large fig; 2 dates, prunes, or plums; 3 apricot halves; 2 tablespoons of raisins or currants; or 12 tart cherries

Fruit Juices

Benefits: Concentrated source of vitamins and antioxidants

Choose: Unsweetened, 100 percent fruit juice concentrates such as tart cherry, blueberry, and pomegranate

Brands: Knudsen, Whole Foods, Lakewood, Eden

Bodily Consumption: 2 to 4 tablespoons

Healthy Sweeteners

Benefits: Smart substitutes for white sugar; provides mineral and antibacterial benefits

Choose: 1 tablespoon date sugar (Bob's Red Mill), brown rice syrup, pure maple syrup, blackstrap molasses (Plantation), or unheated honey; or 2 tablespoons unsweetened 100% fruit preserves (Eden, Bionaturae, Cascadian Farms)

Clean Carbs

Benefit: Gluten-free, hypoallergenic flours and nut meal for baking

Choose from: Buckwheat, garbanzo, quinoa, brown rice, oat meal, and almond meal

Bodily Consumption: ½ cup to be used in baking muffins, cakes, crackers

Special Treats

Cacao Nibs, Cocoa Powder, and Dark, Unsweetened Chocolate

Benefits: High in relaxing magnesium and flavonoids; also high copper sources

Brands: Sunfood Nutrition, TerrAmazon, Dagoba Organic Chocolate, Green & Black, Scharffen Berger

Bodily Consumption: 1 ounce or 1 teaspoon, once per week for baking, yogurt, frappés

FAT FLUSHING FESTIVE MENUS

Winter Vegetarian Buffet for Eight
    Baby Spinach Salad with Daikon Radish
    Sesame Vinaigrette* (page 238)
    Asian Arame Salad* (page 220)
    Cucumber, Wakame, and Tofu Salad* (page 220)
    Szechuan Tofu and Eggplant* (page 221)
    Steamed Baby Carrots with Seaweed Gomasio
    Tart Cherry Kanten* (page 244)
    Apple and Pear Wedges
    Ginger-Honey Yogurt Dip* (page 250)

Romantic Valentine's Dinner for Two
    Beet and Fresh Herbs Salad with Macadamia Nut Oil Vinaigrette* (page 230)
    Tilapia with Spinach-Walnut Pesto* (page 218)
    Roasted Green Beans with Marjoram
    Wilted Red Cabbage with Fennel* (page 227)
    Chocolate Bliss Fondue* (page 245)

Elegant Springtime Dinner with Friends for Eight
    Bitter Greens Salad with Citrus-Infused Vinaigrette* (page 231)
    Pan-Roasted Chicken with Sweet Potatoes* (page 210)
    Sautéed Broccoli Rabe with Shallots
    Quinoa "Risotto"* (page 228)
    Fruit Kebabs with Wild Berry Coulis* (page 239)

Passover Lunch for Eight
    Artichoke and Hearts of Palm Salad* (page 230)
    Poached Salmon with Fresh Herbed Mayonnaise* (page 235)
    Warm Asparagus with Toasted Pine Nuts
    Roasted Baby Red Potatoes with Fresh Dill
    Spelt and Whole Wheat Matzo
    Hungarian Almond Torte* (page 243) with Fresh Whipped Cream
    Array of Fresh Berries

Easter Luncheon for Eight
   Beet and Fresh Herbs Salad with Macadamia Nut Oil Vinaigrette* (page 230)
   Roast Leg of Lamb with Fresh Herbs
   Braised Fragrant Chard* (page 227)
   Jasmine Rice with Green Onions and Bell Peppers
   Sweetie Po' Puffs * (page 240) with Wild Berry Coulis* (page 239)
   Fresh Strawberries, Raspberries, and Blackberries
Summer Breeze Luncheon for Eight
   Chickpea Tahini Pâté* (page 249)
   Fresh Vegetable Crudités
   Poached Salmon with Fresh Herbed Mayonnaise* (page 235) on a Bed of Endive, Watercress, and Radicchio
   Summer Fruit Crumble* (page 242)
   Watermelon Wedges
Fourth of July Barbecue for Eight
   Roasted Eggplant Spread* (page 196)
   Chunky Artichoke Dip* (page 247)
   Veggie Crudités
   Baby Greens Salad with Mediterranean Vinaigrette* (page 238)
   Grilled Chicken
   Grilled Beef Burgers with Lettuce, Tomatoes, and Salsa
   Quick 'n' E-Z Spicy Shrimp* (page 217)
   Veggie Kebabs
   Fresh Pineapple Wedges
Autumn Harvest Brunch for Eight
   Egg and Turkey Bacon Burritos* (page 207)
   Butternut Squashed Fritters* (page 204) with Wild Berry Coulis* (page 239)
   Autumn Fruit Salad with Apples, Pears, and Cranberries
   Warm Apple and Dandelion Root Tea Frappé* (page 202)
   Pumpkin Pie Frappé* (page 202)
Thanksgiving Buffet for Eight
   Bitter Greens Salad with Citrus-Infused Vinaigrette* (page 231)
   Roast Turkey with Sage and Marjoram
   Roasted Pumpkin with Cranberries* (page 229)
   Quinoa Risotto* (page 228)

Braised Fragrant Chard* (page 227)
Array of Seasonal Roasted Vegetables
Fresh Cranberry Chutney* (page 236)
Favorite Pumpkin Pie* (page 243)
Baked Apples

Hanukkah Buffet for Twelve
Chickpea Tahini Pâté* (page 249)
Vegetable Crudités
Beet Borscht* (page 233)
Cinnamon-Scented Cranberry Brisket* (page 214)
Roasted Moroccan Spiced Chicken* (page 209)
Spaghetti Squash Latkes* (page 226) with Applesauce
Roasted Root Veggies * (page 229) with Macadamia Nut Oil Drizzle
Sautéed Green Beans with Mushrooms and Toasted Hazelnuts
Maple-Infused Pears* (page 241)

Christmas Dinner for Eight
Baby Greens and Radicchio with Herbal Dijon Vinaigrette* (page 238)
Curried Delicata Squash Bisque* (page 233)
Roast Beef Tenderloin with Fresh Herbs
Wilted Red Cabbage with Fennel* (page 227)
Orange-Scented Roasted Brussels Sprouts* (page 230)
Roasted Root Veggies* (page 229) with Macadamia Nut Oil Drizzle
Tart Cherry Kanten* (page 244)
Hungarian Almond Torte * (page 243) with Fresh Whipped Cream

New Year's Eve Cocktail Party for Twelve
Persian Meatball and Vegetable Skewers* (page 214)
Crab Cakes in a Flash* (page 216) with Roasted Red Pepper Sauce* (page 236)
Spinach- and Goat Cheese–Stuffed Portobellos* (page 225)
Crunchy Chickpeas* (page 249)
Toasted Tortilla Triangles
Lemony Tapenade* (page 248)
Array of Veggie Crudités
Chunky Artichoke Dip* (page 247)
Fruit Kebabs with Wild Berry Coulis* (page 239)

21 FAT FLUSH FOR LIFE RECIPE COLLECTION

FAT FLUSHING SIGNATURE STAPLES

Cranberry H$_2$O

Homemade Cranberry Juice

Green Life Cocktail

Hot Lemon Water

Spiced Lemon Toddy

Fat Flushing Frappés

Cranberry H$_2$O

My foundational Fat Flushing beverage helps melt away stubborn cellulite and release fluid from waterlogged tissues while detoxifying your liver. It is rather cooling, so don't be afraid to warm it up a bit in the winter and early spring. *Makes 64 ounces*

8 ounces unsweetened cranberry juice, or 3 tablespoons concentrate
56 ounces plain filtered water, or 64 ounces if using cranberry concentrate

In a 64-ounce (½-gallon) bottle, stir together the cranberry juice or concentrate with the water.

Notes from the Fat Flush Kitchen
Allergic to cranberry juice?
Replace 8 ounces of unsweetened cranberry juice with 2 ounces of unsweetened pomegranate juice (POM Wonderful); or omit the cranberry juice and add 4 tablespoons of unfiltered apple cider vinegar to 64 ounces of plain filtered water.
Concerned about plastic bottles?
Check out UNI-KEY's BPA-Free Cran-Water Bottle, which guarantees no plastic or dioxin leaching and no temperature distortion. (See resources.)
For all seasonal Fat Flushes: 64 ounces of Cranberry H$_2$O is your total daily allotment to be divided between the daily Green Life Cocktail and frappés, and taken between meals. Enjoy as much additional plain filtered water as you like.
All Seasons

Homemade Cranberry Juice

This is a fun, easy, and inexpensive way to make your own pure cranberry juice, keeping all the pulp. I often make numerous batches at one time and freeze. If you shop in late December or early January, you can find cranberries for a fraction of their normal price.—Jamie Z., Sandy, Utah
Makes 32 ounces (1 quart)—enough for four days of Cranberry H_2O

1 (12-ounce) bag fresh cranberries
4 cups plain filtered water

Wash the cranberries. Place the berries in a blender with the water. Blend on high speed for 2 to 3 minutes. Pour the cranberry mixture into a saucepan; heat over medium-high heat, being careful not to let the mixture boil. Decrease the heat to medium-low; simmer for about 30 minutes; remove from the heat and let cool. Pour into a container and refrigerate.

Notes from the Fat Flush Kitchen

To make Cranberry H_2O, follow the above recipe using 8 ounces of homemade cranberry juice instead of the 8 ounces of bottled cranberry juice. *All seasons*

Green Life Cocktail

The Green Life Cocktail will purify your system in one green sweep. The added benefits of the probiotic Flora-Key and Cranberry H_2O work together with the greens to clear the path for detoxification. *Makes 1 serving*

1 teaspoon greens powder (pure wheat grass or Liver-Lovin' Formula)
1 teaspoon Flora-Key
8 ounces Cranberry H_2O (page 198)

Stir your choice of greens and Flora-Key into the Cranberry H_2O. Drink up.

Notes from the Fat Flush Kitchen

If you're time-crunched in the morning, make a Fabulous Fat Flush Frappé by adding your greens powder to the blender. *All seasons*

Hot Lemon Water

Sipping this palate-cleansing drink upon arising will gently help to flush your liver and kidneys of accumulated toxins and wastes. *Makes 1 serving*

1 cup hot water
Juice of ½ lemon or lime

Squeeze the lemon into the hot water. Sip slowly.

Notes from the Fat Flush Kitchen

You may substitute 1 tablespoon bottled 100 percent lemon or lime juice (Santa Cruz Organic 100% Lemon or Lime Juice, not from concentrate) for the freshly squeezed lemon or lime juice. For added probiotic punch and a touch of sweetness, let the Hot Lemon Water cool a bit and stir in 1 teaspoon of Flora-Key. This is how we make lemonade out of lemons! *Summer Fat Flush and early Autumn Fat Flush*

Spiced Lemon Toddy

A pinch of aromatic ginger and cinnamon gives your digestion a warming boost to kick-start elimination, especially in the cold weather. *Makes 1 serving*

1 cup hot water   *Pinch of ground ginger*
Juice of ½ lemon   *Pinch of ground cinnamon*

Squeeze the lemon into the hot water; stir in the spices. Sip slowly.

Notes from the Fat Flush Kitchen

If you prefer not to use the spices, you may continue to enjoy this as Hot Lemon Water for Summer and early Autumn Fat Flush.

For an added probiotic punch and a touch of sweetness, let the Spiced Lemon Toddy cool a bit and stir in 1 teaspoon of Flora-Key. *Winter, Spring, and late Autumn Fat Flush*

FAT FLUSHING FRAPPÉS

These deliciously easy-to-prepare frappés will liven up your taste buds with their endless array of fruit combinations. A veteran Fat Flusher once told me she could go for an entire month without making the same frappé twice! Chia seeds provide an unbeatable source of omega-3s as well as soluble fiber, which slows the conversion of carbohydrates into sugar—ideal for those with blood sugar challenges. Best of all, these frappés have the added bonus of keeping you satisfied for up to four hours. These can be frozen as a fun dessert or snack when you need to cool off in the hot summer months.

Basic Fat Flush Frappé

Makes 1 serving

8 ounces Cranberry H_2O (page 198)
1 serving Fat Flush Vanilla Whey
*   Protein or Fat Flush Body Protein*
1 serving fresh or frozen fruit

1 tablespoon flaxseed oil
1 tablespoon chia seeds
1 teaspoon Flora-Key
3 ice cubes, or as desired

Combine the Cranberry H_2O, whey, fruit, flaxseed oil, chia seeds, and Flora-Key in a blender on high speed. Add the ice cubes and continue blending on high speed until the frappé is thick and creamy. Refrigerate or freeze for later use.

Notes from the Fat Flush Kitchen

You may replace the flaxseed oil with 1 tablespoon of lemon-flavored fish oil.

Vegetarian Fat Flushers (or for those who want variety or are sensitive to whey) may choose Fat Flush Body Protein, which is dairy and soy free and made from rice and pea protein.

Chocolate whey protein, a high copper source, is limited to two servings per week. See "Frappé Variations" (pages 201–203) for delicious ways to get your chocolate fix! *All seasons*

Frappé Variations for All Seasons

Blackberry Blast Frappé: use 1 cup of blackberries
Just Cherries Frappé: use 10 large cherries
Berry Wonderful Frappé: use 1 cup of mixed berries
Blushing Peach Frappé: use ½ peach and ½ cup of raspberries
Choco-Cherry Oblivion Frappé: use Fat Flush Chocolate Whey Protein and 10
    large cherries
Rhubarb Berry Burst Frappé: use ½ cup of rhubarb and 6 large strawberries

Blueberry Vanilla Frappé: use 1 cup of blueberries

Strawberry Swirl Frappé: use Fat Flush Chocolate Whey Protein and 6 large strawberries

Blueberry Frappé with a Twist: use 1 cup of blueberries and a squeeze of lime

Peaches 'n' Cream Frappé: use 1 peach

Berries 'n' Cherries Frappé: use 3 large strawberries and 5 large cherries

Raspberry Truffle Frappé: use Fat Flush Chocolate Whey Protein and 1 cup of raspberries

Choco-Rhuberry Frappé: use Fat Flush Chocolate Whey Protein, ½ cup of rhubarb, 3 large strawberries, and ½ cup of raspberries

Pears 'n' Cinnamon Frappé: use 1 pear, ⅛ teaspoon ground cinnamon, and a pinch of ground ginger

Orange Creamsicle Frappé: use the flesh of 1 orange, 2 teaspoons of orange zest, and a pinch of ground ginger

Tootsie Roll Twist Frappé: use ½ serving each of Fat Flush Vanilla and Chocolate Whey Protein, and 6 large strawberries

Strawberry Cream Frappé: use 4 ounces of silken tofu and 6 large strawberries (omit the Fat Flush Whey or Fat Flush Body Protein)

Peach Melba Frappé: use ¼ peach, ¼ cup of raspberries, and the flesh of ½ orange

Hot Mocchachino Frappé: replace the Cranberry H_2O with 8 ounces of hot regular coffee, and omit the Flora-Key and flaxseed oil; sweeten with Stevia Plus, if desired

Frappé Variations for Spring Fat Flush

Warm Apple and Dandelion Root Tea Frappé: use 1 apple, 1 cup of warm dandelion root tea, a 1-inch piece of peeled fresh ginger, and a pinch each of ground cinnamon and cloves

Pumpkin Pie Frappé: use ½ cup of unsweetened pumpkin, 1 apple, ⅛ teaspoon of ground cinnamon, and a pinch each of ground ginger and cloves

Blackberry Mojito Tease Frappé: use 1 cup of blackberries, 2 teaspoons of fresh lime juice, and 2 fresh mint leaves

Blueberry Cheesecake Frappé: use 1 cup of blueberries, ½ cup of cooked butternut squash, and the juice and zest of 1 lime

Frappé Variations for Summer Fat Flush

Amazon Rain Forest Frappé: use ¼ cup of pineapple chunks, ¼ banana, the juice of 1 lime, and 1 tablespoon of flaxseed oil

Frappé Variations for late Autumn and Winter Fat Flush

Wild Berry Crunch Frappé: use ½ cup of blackberries, ¼ cup each of raspberries and blueberries, 7 almonds, ⅛ teaspoon of almond extract, and replace the flaxseed oil with 1 tablespoon of macadamia nut oil

Choco-Banana Frappé: replace the Cranberry H_2O with 8 ounces of plain yogurt; use Fat Flush Chocolate Whey Protein, ½ banana, and ⅛ teaspoon of vanilla extract; and replace the flaxseed oil with 1 tablespoon of coconut oil

Peanut Butter Sundae Frappé: add ½ cup of applesauce, ½ teaspoon of vanilla extract, and 1 tablespoon of peanut butter

Peachy Keene Frappé: replace the Cranberry H_2O with 8 ounces plain kefir; use 1 peach and replace the flaxseed oil with 1 tablespoon of macadamia nut oil

Blueberry Heaven Frappé: replace the Cranberry H_2O with 8 ounces plain yogurt, use ½ cup of blueberries, and replace the flaxseed oil with 1 tablespoon of coconut oil

Raspberry Rapture Frappé: replace the Cranberry H_2O with 8 ounces of plain kefir, use 1 cup of raspberries, and replace the flaxseed oil with 1 tablespoon of macadamia nut oil

BREAKFAST

Pancakes, Cereals, and More
    Spaghetti Squash Pudding
    Blueberry Mini Chiacakes
    Butternut Squashed Fritters
    Break of Dawn Oatmeal

Eggstraordinary Eggs
    Egg, Portobello, and Spinach
    Tower
    Sunshine Frittata
    Mediterranean Scramble
    Egg and Turkey Bacon Burrito

Pancakes, Cereals, and More

Spaghetti Squash Pudding

I created this recipe because I wanted a quick, tasty breakfast or snack I could eat on the go. After posting the original recipe on the Forum, I found many Fat Flushers tweaked the recipe to suit their individual tastes.—Barbara A., Ozark, Arkansas. *Makes 1 to 2 servings*

Olive oil spray
4 large eggs
1 serving Fat Flush Vanilla or Chocolate
    Whey Protein

2 packets Stevia Plus
3 cups cooked spaghetti squash, drained
    well
1 cup fresh or frozen raspberries

Preheat the oven to 350°F. Lightly coat a glass 9-inch pie pan (or an 11 × 7-inch dish) with a few spritzes of olive oil. Mix the eggs on low speed in a blender. Add the whey and Stevia Plus; blend well on low speed. Add the spaghetti squash; blend on high speed until pureed. Sprinkle the raspberries into the pan. Pour the spaghetti squash mixture into the pan. Bake for 25 to 30 minutes, or until set. Chill.

Notes from the Fat Flush Kitchen
Cherries or apples make delicious substitutions for the raspberries. Or, if you prefer, omit the fruit so you can enjoy it later in the day. *All seasons*

Blueberry Mini Chiacakes
Chia seeds add a delightful nutty crunch to these yummy pancakes for kids and grown-ups alike. *Makes 1 serving*

Olive oil spray   *1 serving Fat Flush Vanilla Whey*
1 large egg   *Protein or Fat Flush Body Protein*
2 tablespoons Cranberry H₂O or water   *1 cup blueberries*
1 tablespoon chia seeds   *1 teaspoon Flora-Key*

Lightly coat a medium-size pan with a few spritzes of olive oil. In a medium-size bowl, whisk together all the ingredients except the blueberries and Flora-Key. Gently fold ½ cup of the blueberries into the batter. Heat the pan over medium heat. Using a tablespoon, ladle the chia mixture into the pan. Cook until tiny bubbles form on the surface and the chiacakes are solid enough to turn. Carefully flip the chiacakes, cooking only until done. Transfer to a plate and keep warm. Repeat the process with the remaining batter, coating the pan with a few spritzes of olive oil as needed. Garnish with the remaining ½ cup of blueberries. Sprinkle with the Flora-Key.

Notes from the Fat Flush Kitchen
Blueberries are terrific in these chiacakes, but so are raspberries! Feel free to experiment with other fruits as well, such as apples or pears. *All seasons*

Butternut Squashed Fritters
These fritters are not really squashed at all—rather just a play on words for a pancake made with butternut squash. Best of all—these fritters are not fried but they sure taste like it. *Makes 1 serving*

Olive oil spray

2 tablespoons water

1 apple, peeled, cored, and cut into chunks

¼ teaspoon ground cinnamon

½ cup cooked butternut squash, well drained

1 large egg, beaten

1 serving Fat Flush Vanilla Whey Protein or Fat Flush Body Protein

1 tablespoon chia seeds

1 teaspoon Flora-Key

Spritz a small skillet with olive oil. Add the water to the pan; heat over medium heat. Sauté the apple slices with the cinnamon, stirring constantly, for 1 to 2 minutes, or until softened. In a blender or food processor, blend the apples with the remaining ingredients, except the Flora-Key, until just small chunks remain. Lightly coat the skillet again with a few spritzes of olive oil; heat over medium heat. Ladle the squash mixture into the pan by the heaping tablespoon and cook for about 3 minutes per side, until lightly browned. Carefully flip the fritter, cooking only until done, about 1 minute. Sprinkle with the Flora-Key.

Notes from the Fat Flush Kitchen

Butternut Squashed Fritters are a terrific way to sneak healthy squash into your kid's meals. For a Thanksgiving treat, try replacing the squash with ½ cup of unsweetened pumpkin. *Winter, Spring, and mid-Autumn Fat Flush*

Break of Dawn Oatmeal

This oatmeal is traditionally a cool-weather morning favorite. *Makes 4 servings*

1 cup steel-cut oats

4 cups boiling water

1 crisp apple, peeled, cored, and chopped

½ teaspoon ground cinnamon

¼ teaspoon ground ginger

¼ teaspoon ground nutmeg

Preheat the oven to 200°F. Combine the oats, boiling water, apple, and spices in an ovenproof bowl with a lid. Cover; bake overnight (or at least 8 hours). Or simply place all the ingredients except apples in a small slow cooker. Cook overnight (about 8 hours) on a low setting. Stir in the apples 10 minutes before serving. Sweet dreams!

Notes from the Fat Flush Kitchen

Steel-cut oats, also called whole-grain groats, are actually the inside of the oat kernel, cut into two or three pieces, resembling rice kernels. Other names for steel-cut oats are Irish or Scotch oats. Most people are more familiar with rolled oats. However, for long-cooking oatmeal, steel-cut oats are the appropriate choice. A quarter cup of toasted pecans would be a nice addition. *Winter, late Spring, and mid-Autumn Fat Flush*

Eggstraordinary Eggs

Egg, Portobello, and Spinach Tower

A quick 'n' easy breakfast that contains the filling "umami" factor: the delicious and satisfying portobello mushroom! *Makes 1 serving*

Olive oil spray
1 large egg
Handful of baby spinach
1 slice of red bell pepper

1 medium-size portobello mushroom cap, stem removed
Chopped fresh cilantro
Seaweed Gomasio

Coat a small skillet with a few spritzes of olive oil; heat over medium heat. Break the egg into the pan and cook for about 1 minute. Flip and cook another minute, until the yolk is solid. On a dish, layer the baby spinach and red pepper on top of the mushroom. Top with the cooked egg and chopped cilantro. Sprinkle with Seaweed Gomasio. *All seasons*

Sunshine Frittata

The delicate flavors of artichokes and fresh herbs combine with the earthiness of turkey bacon in this colorful frittata. *Makes 2 servings*

Olive oil spray
1 orange or red bell pepper, seeded and chopped
6 artichoke hearts, chopped
4 large eggs
1 tablespoon water

4 slices turkey bacon, cooked and crumbled
1 tablespoon chopped fresh parsley
1 tablespoon chopped fresh dill
Cayenne

Spritz a medium-size ovenproof skillet with olive oil; heat over medium heat. Sauté the bell pepper and artichokes for 2 minutes. While the veggies are cooking, in medium-size bowl, whisk together the eggs, water, turkey bacon crumbles, herbs, and cayenne to taste. Preheat the broiler. Pour the eggs into the skillet; cook on the stovetop for about 6 minutes, or until top of frittata is set. Place the skillet under the broiler for about 1 minute, or just until the frittata starts to turn golden brown.

Notes from the Fat Flush Kitchen

Make it in autumn by omitting the turkey bacon. In winter, sprinkle the frittata with ¼ cup of shredded cheddar cheese before broiling, if desired. *Winter, Spring, and Summer Fat Flush*

Mediterranean Scramble

Start your day with this easy egg breakfast. Your mornings will seem a little brighter with a taste of Italy. *Makes 1 serving*

Olive oil spray

2 large eggs, beaten

¼ cup chopped asparagus

¼ cup chopped tomato

½ teaspoon dried basil

3 chopped black olives

Pinch of cayenne

Coat a small skillet with a few spritzes of olive oil; heat over medium heat. Whisk together all the ingredients; pour into the pan. Cook for 1 to 2 minutes. Carefully turn over; continue cooking 1 to 2 minutes longer, or until the eggs are set.

Notes from the Fat Flush Kitchen

Try replacing the asparagus and tomato with mushrooms, spinach, zucchini, broccoli, or yellow squash. For Summer Fat Flush, replace the basil with parsley. *Winter, Spring, and late Autumn Fat Flush*

Egg and Turkey Bacon Burrito

This mouth-watering burrito will banish any thoughts of ever stopping for a fast-food breakfast again. *Makes 1 serving*

Olive oil spray

1 large egg

2 slices cooked turkey bacon

1 Ezekiel 4:9 tortilla, warmed

1 tablespoon chopped green onions

2 tablespoons salsa

Coat a small skillet with a few spritzes of oil; heat over medium heat. Place the egg and turkey bacon on the warmed tortilla. Top with the green onions and salsa. Carefully fold in the bottom of the tortilla toward the middle. Then fold in both sides of the tortilla toward the middle.

Notes from the Fat Flush Kitchen

Make it vegetarian by substituting 2 ounces of cooked tempeh strips for the turkey bacon. *Winter and Spring Fat Flush*

LUNCH AND DINNER ENTRÉES

Fowl Play—Chicken and Turkey
   Can't-Resist Chick 'n' Spinach Chili
   1-2-3 Salsa Chicken
   Roasted Moroccan Spiced Chicken
   Chicken Cacciatore
   Pan-Roasted Chicken with Sweet
   Potatoes
   Turkey Scaloppine Skillet Supper

What's Your Beef?
   Effortless Beef Chili
   Cuban Ropa Vieja
   Soft Tacos Olé
   Cinnamon-Scented Cranberry
   Brisket
   Persian Meatball and Vegetable
   Skewers
   Indian Lamb Curry

Fish and Seafood Creations
   Poached Salmon with Fresh
   Herbed Mayonnaise
   Crab Cakes in a Flash
   Quick 'n' E-Z Spicy Shrimp
   Pan-Seared Shrimp with Corn
   Salsa
   Tilapia with Spinach-Walnut Pesto

Entrée Salads
   Dragon Bowl Salad
   Cucumber, Wakame, and Tofu
   Salad
   Asian Arame Salad

Vegetarian Specialties
   Szechuan Tofu and Eggplant
   'Shrooms 'n' Tempeh Chili
   Ethiopian Lentil Stew
   Black Bean Cakes
   Sautéed Escarole with Chickpeas
   Dhal
   Spinach- and Goat Cheese–Stuffed
   Portobellos

Fowl Play: Chicken and Turkey

Can't-Resist Chick 'n' Spinach Chili

I created my Spinach Chili because I needed to eat more greens. The cumin, cilantro, and cayenne are what I like best. In the winter, this chili is a favorite breakfast.—Sue D., Middlevale, New York. *Makes about four 2-cup servings*

Olive oil spray
1¼ pounds ground chicken
2 tablespoons dried parsley
1 to 2 tablespoons ground cumin
2 teaspoons onion powder

1 teaspoon garlic powder
Cayenne
2 (28-ounce) cans whole tomatoes
2 (10-ounce) packages frozen spinach

Coat a large sauté pan with a few spritzes of olive oil; heat over medium-high heat. Brown the ground chicken with the parsley and spices. Add the tomatoes and spinach; bring to a boil, breaking up the spinach. Lower the heat to low. Simmer for approximately 30 minutes, stirring occasionally.

Notes from the Fat Flush Kitchen

Make it in Autumn by substituting 1 pound of extra-firm tofu cubes for the ground chicken. *Winter, Spring, and Summer Fat Flush*

1-2-3 Salsa Chicken (Slow Cooker)

Dinner? Done! This Salsa Chicken is zesty and so very easy to prepare. It's perfect for potlucks and gatherings, and travels well for seasonal feasts and festivities. *Makes about 6 servings*

1 (6-pound) chicken, neck and giblets removed
1 (16-ounce) jar medium-hot salsa

Place the chicken in a large slow cooker. Pour the entire jar of salsa over the chicken; cover. Cook on high for 1 hour. Continue cooking on low for 3 to 4 hours, or until chicken is thoroughly cooked. Transfer the chicken from the slow cooker to a cutting board, reserving the salsa. Carve the chicken as desired. Garnish with the reserved salsa. Serve hot or chilled. *Winter, Spring, and Summer Fat Flush*

Roasted Moroccan Spiced Chicken

This great entrée is packed with enticing and fragrant flavor. *Makes about 6 servings*

Spice Combination	Chicken
1 cinnamon stick, broken into pieces	1 (4-pound) chicken, neck and giblets
8 whole cloves	removed
1 tablespoon coriander seeds	½ cup chopped fresh cilantro
½ teaspoon cayenne	1 lemon, sliced
2 teaspoons cumin seeds	5 cloves garlic, minced
1 teaspoon fennel seeds	1 cup chicken broth

Prepare the Spice Combination
In a small bowl, stir together the spice mixture ingredients.
Prepare the Chicken
Preheat the oven to 350°F. Rub the spices over chicken, coating thoroughly. Stuff the cavity of the chicken with the cilantro, lemon slices, and garlic. If time allows, let the chicken marinate for 30 minutes to develop the flavors. Roast the chicken breast side down for 45 minutes, basting occasionally with chicken

broth. Turn the chicken over and continue to roast basting occasionally, for approximately 1½ hours, or until the thigh temperature reaches 170°F.

Notes from the Fat Flush Kitchen
Toasting spices really enhances the flavor of this dish. Heat a small skillet over low heat. Place the spices in a dry skillet and heat for a minute or so to release their fragrant oils, shaking the pan constantly to avoid scorching. Transfer the spices to a spice grinder, blender, or mortar and pestle, and crush into a powder. *Winter, Spring, and Summer Fat Flush*

Chicken Cacciatore (Slow Cooker)

Chicken Cacciatore is chock-full of ingredients you probably have already on hand. A perfect no-time-to-shop meal. *Makes 4 servings*

1 medium-size onion, chopped coarsely
4 (6-ounce) frozen skinless, boneless chicken breast halves
1 red bell pepper, seeded and cut into large chunks
1 green bell pepper, seeded and cut into large chunks
8 ounces whole cremini mushrooms, quartered
4 cloves garlic, minced
2 bay leaves

1 (6-ounce) can tomato paste
1 (14-ounce) can diced tomatoes
1 (14-ounce) can whole tomatoes, chopped coarsely
1 (28-ounce) can crushed tomatoes
Cayenne
2 teaspoons dried oregano
2 teaspoons dried basil
2 teaspoons fennel seeds

Place the onion in the bottom of the slow cooker. Lay the frozen chicken breasts over the onion. Arrange the peppers, mushrooms, and garlic on top of the chicken. Add the bay leaves, tomato paste, tomatoes, and spices. Cover; cook on high for 1 hour, then cook on low for about 6 hours, or until the chicken and vegetables are thoroughly cooked.

Notes from the Fat Flush Kitchen
In Winter Fat Flush, serve over brown rice or buckwheat or brown rice noodles. *Winter and Spring Fat Flush*

Pan-Roasted Chicken with Sweet Potatoes

Root veggies such as sweet potatoes are delicious and nurturing, especially when cooked in a roasting pan with chicken. *Makes 4 servings*

Olive oil spray
1 lemon, sliced
½ teaspoon grated lemon zest
1 tablespoon freshly squeezed lemon juice
7 cloves garlic, minced

1 teaspoon chopped fresh oregano, or ¼
    teaspoon dried
8 skinless chicken thighs
12 black olives
4 small sweet potatoes, peeled, quartered,
    and sliced

Preheat the oven to 425°F. Coat a large roasting pan with a few spritzes of olive oil. Layer the slices of lemon in bottom of pan. In a large bowl, stir together the lemon zest, lemon juice, four cloves' worth of the minced garlic, and the oregano. Add the chicken; toss to coat. Arrange the chicken in a single layer on top of the lemon slices. In a medium-size bowl, combine the olives, sweet potatoes, and the remaining minced garlic; toss to coat. Arrange the sweet potato mixture over the chicken. Bake for 40 to 45 minutes, or until the chicken is cooked through and the sweet potatoes are soft. *Winter and Spring Fat Flush*

Turkey Scaloppine Skillet Supper
This light dish is ready in a flash and is perfect for a quick midweek family dinner. *Makes 4 servings*

Olive oil spray
1¼ pounds turkey breast fillets (can also
    use chicken)
½ cup chicken broth

1 cup sliced onions
2 cups sliced mushrooms
¼ cup minced fresh parsley, plus extra
    for garnish

Lightly coat a large skillet with a few spritzes of olive oil; heat over medium heat. Sauté the turkey until browned and almost cooked through. Transfer to a plate and keep warm. Heat the broth in the skillet and sauté the onions and mushrooms until nicely browned. Return the turkey to the pan. Stir in the minced parsley; continue heating until bubbly and the turkey is cooked through. Sprinkle with additional minced parsley.

Notes from the Fat Flush Kitchen
For a change of tastes and textures, try a variety of mushrooms such as shiitake, cremini, and portobellos. A pinch of Seaweed Gomasio adds a nice flavor punch. *Winter, Spring, and Summer Fat Flush*

What's Your Beef?

Effortless Beef Chili (Slow Cooker)

This recipe was all about convenience—tossing everything in the slow cooker and coming home from work to find tasty chili. The only work needed was to break up the meat with a fork and eat.—Charli S., Beverly, Washington *Makes about four 2-cup servings*

2 onions, sliced

1¼ pounds frozen lean ground meat

1 cup sliced mushrooms

1 (6-ounce) can tomato paste

1 (28-ounce) can diced tomatoes

2 to 3 garlic cloves, minced

2 teaspoon ground cumin

Cayenne

1 bay leaf

Place the onions in the bottom of the slow cooker. Place the frozen ground meat over the onions. Lay the mushrooms on top of the ground meat. In a small bowl, mix together the remaining ingredients; pour over the mushrooms. Cover; cook on low for 6 to 8 hours (or on high for 4 to 5 hours). About 45 minutes prior to serving, use a wooden spoon to break apart the meat into small chunks. Remove and discard the bay leaf before serving. *Winter, Spring, and Summer Fat Flush*

Cuban Ropa Vieja (Stove or Slow Cooker)

A flank steak twist with Caribbean-style spices, one of our all-time Fat Flushing favorites. *Makes about eight 2-cup servings*

Olive oil spray

2½ pounds flank steak, cut crosswise into
    three pieces

2 large onions, sliced thinly

2 bell peppers (any color), sliced thinly
    and seeded

3 cloves garlic, minced

2 tablespoons apple cider vinegar

2 cups beef broth

1 (14-ounce) can diced tomatoes

2 bay leaves

2 tablespoons ground cumin

1 to 2 jalapeños, chopped

2 tablespoons tomato paste

Prepare on the Stove

Lightly coat a large pot with a few spritzes of olive oil; heat over high heat. Brown the meat on all sides, approximately 5 minutes. Transfer the meat to a plate. Spritz the pot again; heat over medium-high heat. Add the onions, peppers, and garlic, stirring until they begin to brown. Add the vinegar; stir, scraping up any brown bits from bottom of the pan. Add the broth and diced tomatoes. Bring to a boil over high heat. Add the bay leaves, cumin, jalapeños, and tomato paste, stirring until all the ingredients are blended. Return the steak to the pot. Bring the mixture back up to a boil, cover; lower the heat and simmer until the meat is very tender. This will take approximately 2½ hours. When the meat is tender, shred gently with a fork. Remove and discard the bay leaves before serving.

Prepare in a Slow Cooker

Lightly coat a large sauté pan with a few spritzes of olive oil, heat over high heat. Brown the meat on all sides, approximately 5 minutes. Transfer the meat to the slow cooker. Add the remaining ingredients. Cook on low for about 6 hours, or until very tender. When the meat is tender, shred gently with a fork. Remove and discard the bay leaves before serving. *Winter, Spring, and Summer Fat Flush*

Soft Tacos Olé

Comfort food, Fat Flush–style. *Makes 4 servings*

Olive oil spray
1 onion, chopped
1 red bell pepper, seeded and chopped
1¼ pounds lean ground beef or turkey
3 cloves garlic, chopped
2 teaspoons Fat Flush Seasoning (page 235)

4 Ezekiel 4:9 tortillas, warmed
¼ cup salsa
Chopped green onions and fresh cilantro, for garnish

Coat a large skillet with a few spritzes of olive oil; heat over medium-high heat. Sauté the onions and peppers until softened. Add the ground beef and garlic and continue sautéing until the beef is cooked through; drain. Stir in the Fat Flush Seasoning; simmer for 5 minutes. Spoon the taco mixture into the warmed tortillas; top each with 1 tablespoon of salsa, green onions, and cilantro.

Notes from the Fat Flush Kitchen

For the first month of Summer Fat Flush, omit the tortilla and serve the taco mixture over mixed greens. *Winter, Spring, and mid-Summer Fat Flush*

Cinnamon-Scented Cranberry Brisket

This brisket has graced many a holiday table in my home. I have found that the trick for rich and aromatic gravy is pureeing part of the veggies and juices from the brisket.—Linda S., Naples, Florida. *Makes about 8 servings*

Olive oil spray
3 pounds lean beef brisket, trimmed
1 (12-ounce) bag fresh cranberries,
   picked over and washed
1 large onion, sliced
2 sweet potatoes, peeled and cut into
   chunks
6 cloves garlic, crushed

4 stalks celery, sliced
6 carrots, peeled and sliced
4 whole cinnamon sticks
1 teaspoon dried rosemary
1 teaspoon dried basil
Cayenne
1½ cups beef broth

Preheat the oven to 425°F. Coat a roasting pan with a few spritzes of olive oil; lay the brisket in the pan. Arrange the cranberries, onions, sweet potatoes, garlic, celery, carrots, and cinnamon sticks around the outside edges of brisket. Sprinkle with the rosemary, basil, and cayenne. Roast, uncovered, for 30 minutes. Lower the oven temperature to 300°F. Pour the beef broth over the brisket. Seal the pan tightly on all sides with foil. Roast for 3 hours, or until the brisket is fork-tender. Discard the cinnamon sticks. Place about half the veggies, cranberries, and juices in a blender or food processor; puree on low speed. (Puree in batches if needed.) Pour the gravy over the brisket. Let cool; then refrigerate for at least 8 hours or overnight. (Briskets are much easier to slice when cold.) Slice the brisket thinly and return to the pan to soak in the gravy. Heat the brisket in a gentle oven (about 250°F) until hot, about 25 minutes. *Winter and Spring Fat Flush*

Persian Meatball and Vegetable Skewers

Deliciously different but guaranteed to please, these beef and pepper skewers are completely transformed by the exotic spices. You will need eight 10- to 12-inch skewers; if using wood or bamboo, soak in water for 30 minutes before threading with the kebabs. *Makes 4 servings*

1¼ pounds lean ground beef (do not use
   extra-lean)
1 large egg
3 green onions, minced
¼ cup chopped fresh parsley

¼ cup chopped fresh cilantro
¼ teaspoon ground ginger
¼ teaspoon ground cloves
¼ teaspoon ground cinnamon
1 teaspoon ground cumin

1 teaspoon ground coriander

2 cloves garlic, minced

3 tablespoons tomato sauce

1 orange bell pepper

1 red bell pepper

1 green bell pepper

1 onion

½ pound mushrooms (button or cremini)

In a large bowl, mix together the ground beef, egg, green onions, parsley, cilantro, spices, garlic, and tomato sauce. Form the beef mixture into sixteen equal-size oval meatballs. Cut the peppers and onion into chunks approximately 1 inch across. Alternate the meatballs and vegetables on the skewers, beginning and ending with vegetables (four meatballs to a skewer). Grill until the meatballs are cooked through, with no pink remaining, and the vegetables are slightly charred.

Notes from the Fat Flush Kitchen

The meatballs and vegetables can be cooked without the skewers in a grill pan in the broiler or on top of the stove. Bake for 15 minutes, or until the meatballs are cooked through, with no pink remaining. Ground lamb may be used instead of ground beef. For party hors d'oeuvres, use 6-inch skewers. *Winter, Spring and Summer Fat Flush*

Indian Lamb Curry

Why not introduce this flavorful dish year round? *Makes about eight 2-cup servings*

Olive oil spray

3 pounds boneless leg of lamb, trimmed
    and cut into 1-inch pieces

¼ cup beef broth

2 onions, chopped

2 cloves garlic, chopped

2 bay leaves

¼ teaspoon cayenne

2 tablespoons peeled and minced fresh
    ginger

2 teaspoons Garam Masala* (page 234)

½ teaspoon turmeric

½ teaspoon salt (optional)

1 cinnamon stick

4 plum tomatoes, chopped, or 1 (14-
    ounce) can diced tomatoes

1½ cups water

1 cup fresh chopped cilantro

Coat a Dutch oven or deep skillet with a lid with a few spritzes of olive oil; heat over medium-high heat. Sauté the lamb on all sides until browned, about 5 minutes; remove from the pan. Heat the beef broth in the pan over medium-high heat until bubbly. Sauté the onions and garlic for about 5 minutes, or until softened and lightly browned. Stir in the remaining ingredients (including the lamb) except the tomatoes, water, and cilantro; simmer for 5 minutes. Add the tomatoes and water; lower the heat to low, and cover. Simmer the stew for about 1 hour, or until lamb is fork-tender. Before serving, remove the cinnamon stick and bay leaves; stir in the cilantro. *Winter, Spring, and Summer Fat Flush*

Fish and Seafood Creations

Poached Salmon with Fresh Herbed Mayonnaise

Omega-rich poached salmon exudes simple elegance. Nothing looks more inviting at a springtime brunch than fresh salmon when garnished with sprigs of fresh herbs and lemon slices. *Makes 4 servings*

Poaching Liquid
    8 cups water or fish stock
    1 carrot, sliced
    2 shallots, sliced
    1 stalk celery, sliced
    2 lemons, sliced
    4 sprigs fresh dill
    4 sprigs fresh parsley

Salmon
    1 pound salmon fillet
    ½ cup Fresh Herbed Mayonnaise
    (page 235)
    4 sprigs fresh dill
    4 sprigs fresh parsley
    1 lemon, sliced

Prepare the Poaching Liquid
Place all the poaching ingredients in a large deep skillet with a lid. Bring the liquid to a gentle boil; reduce to simmer.
Prepare the Salmon
Add the salmon to the poaching liquid; cover. Maintaining a simmer, poach for 8 to 10 minutes, or until the salmon is opaque and flakes easily with a fork. Place the salmon on a serving plate; refrigerate for at least an hour or until thoroughly chilled. Before serving, carefully slice the salmon into four fillets; top each with 2 tablespoons of Fresh Herbed Mayonnaise. Garnish with sprigs of fresh dill and parsley and lemon slices. *Winter, Spring, and Summer Fat Flush*

Crab Cakes in a Flash

These crab cakes are ideal for time-crunched schedules, no matter what time of year. *Makes 4 servings*

Olive oil spray
1 pound crabmeat, picked over, rinsed,
    and drained
½ medium-size onion, chopped

2 tablespoons seeded and chopped bell
    pepper
2 tablespoons chopped celery
2 tablespoons chopped fresh dill

2 tablespoons chopped fresh parsley
1 clove garlic, minced
Pinch of cayenne

1 tablespoon freshly squeezed lemon or
lime juice
1 large egg, beaten

Preheat the oven to 350°F. Lightly coat a baking sheet with a few spritzes of olive oil. In a large bowl, break up the crabmeat with a fork. Mix in the rest of the ingredients. Shape the mixture into eight patties. Place the patties on the baking sheet. Bake the crab cakes for about 15 minutes, or until nicely browned and cooked through.

Notes from the Fat Flush Kitchen

If time permits, make up the patties in the morning and just pop them in the oven when you get home. For cocktail-size crab cakes, make sixteen instead of eight. *Winter, Spring, and Summer Fat Flush*

Quick 'n' E-Z Spicy Shrimp

Sassy shrimp goes with a medley of your favorite veggies or on top of tossed greens. *Makes 4 servings*

Marinade
Juice of 2 limes
2 cloves garlic, chopped
½ teaspoon ground cumin
Cayenne

Shrimp
1¼ pounds medium raw shrimp,
peeled and tails left on
Olive oil spray

Prepare the Marinade
Combine all the marinade ingredients in a large baking dish. Add the shrimp; toss to coat. Refrigerate the shrimp for 15 minutes.
Prepare the Shrimp
Lightly coat a broiler pan with a few spritzes of olive oil. Broil the shrimp for approximately 3 minutes, or until just pink, occasionally basting with the marinade. Do not overcook. Discard any leftover marinade.

Notes from the Fat Flush Kitchen

The shrimp can also be grilled on skewers. This marinade also works well with scallops. *Winter, Spring, and Summer Fat Flush*

Pan-Seared Shrimp with Corn Salsa

Simple shrimp is jazzed up with the bright flavor of corn salsa. *Makes 4 servings*

Salsa
  2 cups corn
  Juice from 1 lime
  1 small red onion, diced
  1 jalapeño, seeded and chopped finely
  (or more if you like)
  ¼ cup chopped fresh cilantro
  ⅛ teaspoon salt (optional)
  3 tomatoes, seeded and diced

Shrimp
  1 pound large raw shrimp, peeled,
  tails left on
  Salt (optional)
  Cayenne
  2 tablespoons olive oil
  ¼ cup chopped fresh parsley

Prepare the Salsa

In a large bowl, toss together all the salsa ingredients. Refrigerate the salsa for at least 1 hour to allow the flavors to blend.

Prepare the Shrimp

Before serving, season the shrimp lightly on both sides with salt (optional) and cayenne. In a large sauté pan, heat the olive oil over medium-high heat until very hot but not smoking. Add the shrimp; sear on each side for about 2 minutes, or until golden and cooked through. Be careful not to overcook. Divide the shrimp among serving plates; top with equal amounts of salsa and chopped parsley. *Winter Fat Flush*

Tilapia with Spinach-Walnut Pesto

Nutty spinach-walnut pesto gives a little pizzazz to the mild-tasting tilapia. Great for a romantic dinner for two. *Makes 4 servings*

Pesto
  1 (3-ounce) package baby spinach
  leaves
  ¼ cup olive oil
  16 walnut halves, toasted
  2 to 4 ounces grated Romano cheese
  1 clove garlic, chopped

Tilapia
  Olive oil spray

  1 (3-ounce) package baby spinach
  leaves
  1 pound tilapia fillets (4 large or 8 small)
  Salt (optional)
  Cayenne
  Juice of 1 lemon
  ¼ cup seeded and chopped red bell
  pepper
  ¼ cup seeded and chopped orange
  bell pepper

Prepare the Pesto

Place all the pesto ingredients in a food processor or blender; pulse, using on and off turns of the switch until well blended.

Prepare the Tilapia

Preheat the oven to 400°F. Lightly coat a 9 × 13-inch baking pan with a few spritzes of olive oil. Scatter the spinach over the bottom of the pan. Sprinkle the fillets on both sides with salt (optional) and cayenne. Layer the tilapia fillets on top of the spinach. Drizzle the fillets with lemon juice. Spread an equal amount of pesto on top of each fillet. Scatter the chopped peppers over the fillets. Bake for about 15 minutes, or until the fillets are opaque and flake easily with a fork.

Notes from the Fat Flush Kitchen

Toast the walnuts on a baking sheet at 350°F for 7 to 10 minutes, or until golden brown, shaking pan occasionally. Or toast in a dry skillet over medium heat for 7 to 10 minutes, shaking the pan constantly. Be careful not to burn. Let cool. *Winter Fat Flush*

Entrée Salads

Dragon Bowl Salad

This hearty salad is healthy and utterly satisfying. *Makes 1 serving*

2 cups mixed salad greens

1 medium-size tomato, seeded and cut into wedges

¼ cup chopped cucumber

¼ cup chopped, mixed fresh parsley, cilantro, and dill

1 tablespoon chopped onion

½ cup cauliflower florets

½ cup broccoli florets

4 canned artichoke hearts, quartered

2 hearts of palm, sliced

1 stalk celery, chopped

3 baby carrots, sliced

3 sliced olives

4 ounces of beef, chicken, turkey, fish, seafood, tofu, or tempeh

Dressing of choice

Combine all the herbs and vegetables in a large bowl. Toss the salad with your protein food and dressing of choice.

Notes from the Fat Flush Kitchen

Take advantage of all the colorful veggies your local farmers' market has to offer, such as arugula, yellow squash, and zucchini. *All seasons*

Cucumber, Wakame, and Tofu Salad

You'll flip for this light sea veggie salad. Each ingredient has a distinct texture and flavor of its own. *Makes about four 2-cup servings*

Salad
  ½ cup wakame
  1 pound firm tofu, cut into cubes
  2 cucumbers, peeled and sliced into
  1-inch rounds
  ½ cup sliced water chestnuts
  2 green onions, chopped finely

Dressing
  ¼ cup flaxseed oil
  2 tablespoons apple cider vinegar
  1 teaspoon Seaweed Gomasio

Prepare the Salad

Soak the wakame in water for 15 minutes; drain, rinse, and chop coarsely. In a medium-size bowl, stir the wakame with the remaining ingredients.

Prepare the Dressing

In a measuring cup, blend the dressing ingredients; toss with the vegetables. Let stand at room temperature for 15 minutes prior to serving, to allow the flavors to blend.

Notes from the Fat Flush Kitchen

In Winter Fat Flush, substitute sesame oil for the flaxseed oil, for a subtle Asian flavor. *All seasons*

Asian Arame Salad

This unique summer salad, featuring arame, tofu, and daikon, delivers high-level nutrition. *Makes about four 2-cup servings*

2 cups arame, soaked and drained

Dressing
  2 cloves garlic, minced
  1½ teaspoons grated fresh ginger
  ¼ cup apple cider vinegar
  2 tablespoons sesame oil
  ½ teaspoon Seaweed Gomasio

Salad
  16 ounces firm tofu, cubed
  ½ cup diced carrots, steamed and
  drained
  1 red bell pepper, seeded and cut into
  strips
  3 green onions, sliced
  1 (4-inch) piece daikon radish, grated
  2 tablespoons toasted sesame seeds

Prepare the Dressing
Combine all the dressing ingredients in a jar with a lid; shake well.
Prepare the Salad
Place the soaked and drained arame in a large bowl. Add the salad ingredients.
Toss the arame and salad ingredients with the dressing mixture. Refrigerate for
30 minutes prior to serving, to allow flavors to blend.

Notes from the Fat Flush Kitchen
To soak arame, place in a saucepan of hot water for 15 minutes; drain.
For feasts and festivities, try adding 1 tablespoon of wheat-free tamari to the
dressing. *Winter and late Autumn Fat Flush*

Vegetarian Specialties

Szechuan Tofu and Eggplant
Hot and spicy, this dish will awaken your senses with the flavors of Asia. Not for
mild-mannered taste buds. *Makes about four 2-cup servings*

Olive oil spray
2 large eggplants, peeled and cut into
*   chunks*
2 onions, chopped
4 stalks celery, sliced
2 red and/or green bell peppers, seeded
*   and cut into chunks*
2 cups vegetable broth
¼ cup freshly squeezed lemon juice

1 (1-inch) piece peeled fresh ginger,
*   minced*
3 cloves garlic, minced
16 ounces extra-firm tofu, cut into
*   chunks*
4 sheets nori, broken into pieces
Cayenne
1 tablespoon Seaweed Gomasio

Lightly coat a large skillet or wok with a few spritzes of olive oil; heat over
medium-high heat. Stir-fry the vegetables until softened, 7 to 10 minutes. Stir in
the broth, lemon juice, ginger, and garlic; heat until bubbly. Add the tofu, nori,
the cayenne to taste, and the Seaweed Gomasio; simmer for about 5 minutes, or
until the nori is softened. *All seasons*

'Shrooms 'n' Tempeh Chili

This chili is mighty tempting and filling...and *not* just for vegetarians. *Makes about four 2-cup servings*

2 (8-ounce) packages plain tempeh
2 (14-ounce) cans diced tomatoes
1 onion, chopped
3 stalks celery, chopped
4 cloves garlic, minced
2 teaspoons ground cumin
1 teaspoon ground coriander
⅛ teaspoon ground cloves

¼ teaspoon cayenne
2 jalapeños, diced (or more if you like)
3 tablespoons apple cider vinegar
½ cup chopped fresh cilantro
½ cup chopped fresh parsley
1 cup vegetable broth
8 ounces mushrooms, quartered

In a large soup pot set over medium heat, stir together all the ingredients except the mushrooms. Bring the mixture to a boil; lower the heat and cover. Simmer, stirring occasionally, for about 45 minutes, or until the veggies are fork-tender. Add the mushrooms; simmer for an additional 10 minutes.

Notes from the Fat Flush Kitchen

For a meaty texture, try portobello or cremini mushrooms. This chili is wonderful served over spaghetti squash or shredded zucchini in Summer Fat Flush. Or try buckwheat (soba) noodles or brown rice pasta in Winter Fat Flush. *All seasons*

Ethiopian Lentil Stew

This enticing lentil stew is packed with North African flavors that will have your family begging for more. *Makes about four 2-cup servings*

Spice Combination
   1 tablespoon coriander
   1 tablespoon ground cloves
   2 teaspoons ground cinnamon
   ½ teaspoon ground ginger
   1 teaspoon garlic powder
   1 tablespoon turmeric
   1 bay leaf
   1 teaspoon cayenne, or to taste
   1 teaspoon salt (optional)

Stew
   1 cup dried red lentils
   2 cups vegetable broth, plus extra if needed
   2 cloves garlic, crushed
   1 to 2 tablespoons Spice Combination (see left column)
   1 (28-ounce) can crushed tomatoes

Prepare the Spices

In a small bowl, stir together all the spices. Place in a covered container or shaker bottle. Store the spices at room temperature away from the stove.

Prepare the Stew

In a medium-size stockpot, mix together the lentils, veggie broth, garlic, and 1 to 2 tablespoons of the spices (save the rest for another use.) Cook the lentil mixture over medium-low heat for about 20 minutes or until the lentils begin to soften. If the lentils start to dry out, add about ½ cup additional veggie broth. Stir in the tomatoes; cover and simmer for about 15 minutes, until lentils are softened and the flavors are combined. Remove and discard the bay leaf before serving. *Mid-Winter and Autumn Fat Flush*

Black Bean Cakes

Bean cakes whip up in no time for a fast nourishing dish. A great protein- and fiber-packed snack to keep the cravings at bay. *Makes 8 servings*

Olive oil spray
½ cup chopped red onion
¼ cup chopped celery
¼ cup seeded and chopped red bell pepper
¼ cup seeded and chopped green bell pepper
2 cloves garlic, minced
1 jalapeño, seeded and chopped
2 teaspoons freshly squeezed lime juice

⅛ teaspoon cayenne, or to taste
1 teaspoon ground cumin
¼ teaspoon ground coriander
1 tablespoon dried parsley
¼ teaspoon salt (optional)
2 (14-ounce) cans black beans, drained and lightly mashed
1 large egg
¼ cup chia seeds

Preheat the oven to 375°F. Coat a sauté pan with a few spritzes of olive oil; heat over medium heat. Sauté the veggies until they are softened and begin to brown, spoon into a large bowl. Stir in the remaining ingredients, mixing well. Form the mixture into eight equal-size patties. Lightly coat a baking sheet with a few spritzes of olive oil. Place the patties on the baking sheet and bake for about 15 minutes, or until heated through. *Mid-Winter and Autumn Fat Flush*

Sautéed Escarole with Chickpeas

Escarole is as delicious as it versatile. Great in stews, stir-fries, soups, and salads. The addition of chickpeas is a healthy twist. *Makes about four 2-cup servings*

2 heads escarole, washed and chopped
   coarsely
Olive oil spray
3 cloves garlic, crushed
2 cups chopped fresh parsley
1 (14-ounce) can chickpeas (garbanzos),
   rinsed and drained

2 tablespoons vegetable broth
2 tablespoons freshly squeezed lemon
   juice
⅛ teaspoon cayenne, or to taste
Pinch of salt (optional)

In a large pot with a lid, lightly steam the escarole till just tender, about 6 minutes; drain. Lightly coat the same pot with a few spritzes of olive oil; heat over medium heat. Sauté the garlic for about 1 minute, or until softened and just beginning to turn golden. Be careful not to burn. Add the escarole, parsley, and chickpeas; sauté for 2 minutes. Stir in the veggie broth, lemon juice, cayenne, and salt (if using). Continue sautéing for about 5 minutes, until escarole is tender and almost all the broth has evaporated.

Notes from the Fat Flush Kitchen

If you have haven't used your oil allowance for the day, a tablespoon of flaxseed oil drizzled on top of the finished dish would be delicious. *Mid-Winter and Autumn Fat Flush*

Dhal (Slow Cooker)

Spiced lentils make an unusually flavorful currylike dish. This is not your mother's version of baked beans. *Makes about four 2-cup servings*

1¼ cups dried lentils, washed and
   drained
2 bay leaves
6 whole cloves
2 cups boiling water
1 onion, chopped coarsely
3 cloves garlic, crushed
1 green bell pepper, seeded and chopped
   coarsely
¼ cup vegetable broth

½ teaspoon ground cinnamon
½ teaspoon ground ginger, or 1 teaspoon
   grated fresh
1 teaspoon turmeric
1 teaspoon ground coriander
Cayenne
½ teaspoon salt (optional)
Juice of 1 lime
1 cup chopped fresh cilantro, with stems

Place the lentils, bay leaves, and cloves in the slow cooker; cover with the boiling water. Stir in remaining ingredients except the lime juice and cilantro. Cook on high for 2 to 2 ½ hours, or until the lentils are tender and the water has been absorbed. Stir in the lime juice and cilantro. Remove and discard the bay leaves before serving.

Notes from the Fat Flush Kitchen

Any type of lentil makes a delicious dhal—red, green yellow, black, or brown. Some markets even have pink, white, and reddish-brown lentils. If you prefer a souplike consistency rather than a stew, cook the lentils until tender with some liquid remaining.

Dhal is delicious served over steamed spinach or brown rice in mid-Winter or late Autumn Fat Flush. *Mid-Winter and Autumn Fat Flush*

Spinach- and Goat Cheese–Stuffed Portobellos

Hits the spot as a light lunch or dinner or even as a quick 'n' easy party hors d'oeuvre. A perennial favorite. *Makes 4 servings*

Olive oil spray

Filling
  ¼ cup vegetable broth
  ½ cup chopped onions
  ½ cup seeded and chopped red bell peppers
  2 teaspoons Fat Flush Seasoning (page 235)

8 cups baby spinach, or three (3-ounce) packages
1 large egg white
¼ cup chia seeds

Mushrooms
  8 medium-size portobello mushroom caps, stems removed
  4 ounces goat cheese, crumbled

Preheat the oven to 375°F. Lightly coat a baking sheet with a few spritzes of olive oil.
Prepare the Filling
In a medium-size skillet, heat the broth over medium heat. Sauté the onions, peppers, and Fat Flush Seasoning in the broth for about 5 minutes, or until the veggies are tender and begin to brown. Stir in the spinach; cook just until the spinach wilts, about 1 minute. Remove the veggies from the heat; stir in the egg white and chia seeds.
Prepare the Mushrooms
Mound the filling equally into the mushroom caps. Sprinkle the mushroom caps with equal portions of the goat cheese. Bake for 15 minutes, or until the mushrooms are heated through and the cheese is melted. *Winter and Autumn Fat Flush*

A POTPOURRI OF VEGETABLES

Side Dishes
  Spaghetti Squash Latkes
  (Pancakes)
  Wilted Red Cabbage with Fennel
  Braised Fragrant Chard
  Baked Parsnip Fries
  Quinoa "Risotto"
  Roasted Pumpkin with
  Cranberries
  Roasted Root Veggies

Orange-Scented Roasted Brussels
Sprouts
Sumptuous Side Salads
  Artichoke and Hearts of Palm
  Salad
  Beet and Fresh Herbs Salad with
  Macadamia Nut Oil Vinaigrette
  Bitter Greens Salad with Citrus-
  Infused Vinaigrette

Side Dishes

Spaghetti Squash Latkes (Pancakes)

It seems there is no end to the versatility of spaghetti squash. If you're cooking one, you might as well cook an extra or two for quick 'n easy dishes throughout the week. Here's one of my family's favorites.—Linda S., Naples, Florida. *Makes 1 serving*

Olive oil spray
2 cups cooked spaghetti squash
1 large egg

⅛ teaspoon ground cinnamon
⅛ teaspoon ground ginger
1 tablespoon chia seeds

Lightly coat a sauté pan with a few spritzes of olive oil and heat over medium heat. In medium-size bowl, mix the cooked spaghetti squash with the egg, cinnamon, ginger, and chia seeds. Ladle about 2 tablespoons of the squash mixture into the pan; cook until small bubbles form on the surface of the pancake. Flip the pancakes over and continue cooking until almost dry. Repeat with the remaining batter.

Notes from the Fat Flush Kitchen
These latkes also make a delicious breakfast or snack. Try replacing the cinnamon and ginger with savory seasonings such as coriander or cumin. *All seasons*

Wilted Red Cabbage with Fennel

A warm slaw that is surprisingly satisfying and easy on your tummy. A nice addition to a late summer or autumn menu. *Makes about four 1-cup servings*

4 cups shredded red cabbage
¼ cup vegetable broth

1 tablespoon apple cider vinegar
1 teaspoon fennel seeds

In medium-size sauté pan, stir-fry the cabbage in the broth over medium-high heat until wilted. Stir in the apple cider vinegar. Continue stir-frying for about 5 minutes, until the juices are reduced. Toss with the fennel seeds. *All seasons*

Braised Fragrant Chard

A spectacularly healthy veggie that is a nutritional powerhouse and tastes good, too. *Makes about four 1-cup servings*

¾ cup vegetable broth
1 onion, chopped
3 cloves garlic, smashed

1 bunch green chard, chopped coarsely
Salt (optional)

In a large sauté pan over medium-high heat, heat ¼ cup of the broth. Sauté the onions and garlic until softened, about 2 minutes. Stir in the chard. Stir in the remaining ½ cup of broth; cover. Lower the heat to low; simmer until the chard is crisp-tender, about 5 minutes. Sprinkle with salt if using.

Notes from the Fat Flush Kitchen

Look for rainbow chard at your local farmers' market or supermarket; it is characterized by its beautiful red and yellow stems. In Winter or late Autumn Fat Flush, try tossing the chard with 1 tablespoon of toasted chopped walnuts. *All seasons*

Baked Parsnip Fries

Unusually nutty and sweet, parsnips are the perfect baked alternative to white potato french fries. *Makes about four ½-cup servings*

1 large egg white
2 teaspoons Fat Flush Seasoning (page 235)
8 parsnips, peeled and cut into "fries"

Preheat the oven to 425°F. Line a baking sheet with parchment paper. In a large bowl, whisk the egg white with the Fat Flush Seasoning until foamy. Toss the parsnips in the egg white mixture until coated. Spread the fries evenly on the baking sheet. Bake for 15 minutes; turn the fries over and bake for 10 to 15 minutes longer, or until browned.

Notes from the Fat Flush Kitchen

This recipe also works well for sweet potatoes and rutabagas. *Winter, Spring, and mid-Autumn Fat Flush*

Quinoa "Risotto"

Quinoa is the substitute of choice for wheat-sensitive individuals. Its nutty, light flavor is very inviting and a perfect complement to spring and summer meals. *Makes about eight ½-cup servings*

2 tablespoons extra-virgin olive oil
1 red bell pepper, seeded and diced
1 onion, diced
1 cup quinoa, rinsed and drained

2 cups vegetable broth, plus extra as
  needed
½ teaspoon salt (optional)

In medium-size saucepan, heat 1 tablespoon of the olive oil over medium heat. Add the peppers and onions; cook until the peppers are soft and the onions are golden, about 10 minutes. (Add some broth if needed to keep the onions from sticking.) Transfer the vegetables to a bowl. Heat the remaining tablespoon of oil in the saucepan. Add the quinoa; cook over medium heat, stirring, until lightly toasted, about 5 minutes. Add the broth and salt, if using; bring to a boil. Cover and simmer until the broth is absorbed and the quinoa is tender, 15 to 20 minutes. Fluff with a fork; stir in the reserved onions and peppers.

Notes from the Fat Flush Kitchen

Quinoa (pronounced *keen wah*) contains a bitter-tasting coating. Before cooking, rinse well in a strainer. *Mid-Winter, mid-Spring, and late Autumn Fat Flush*

Roasted Pumpkin with Cranberries

A nice autumnal side, pumpkin is a high antioxidant veggie that lends itself well to aromatic spices and colorful berries. *Makes about four ½-cup servings*

Olive oil spray

1 small pumpkin (about 3 pounds)

1 teaspoon ground cinnamon

½ teaspoon ground ginger

½ teaspoon ground nutmeg

¼ teaspoon ground cloves

1 cup fresh or frozen cranberries

Preheat the oven to 400°F. Coat a 9 × 11-inch baking dish with a few spritzes of olive oil. In a large bowl, toss together the pumpkin, oil, spices, and cranberries; pour into the baking dish. Spritz lightly with olive oil and bake for about 30 minutes, or until the pumpkin is soft.

Notes from the Fat Flush Kitchen

"Pie" or "sugar" pumpkins provide the best flavor. To remove the flesh from the pumpkin, cut into quarters with a very sharp knife, removing the seeds. Save the seeds for toasting. Carefully cut away the outer shell; cut the flesh into 2-inch chunks. *Winter and mid-Autumn Fat Flush*

Roasted Root Veggies

Root veggies are so sweet when roasted you may want to consider them "dessert," especially in the colder months when they are in season. *Makes about four ½-cup servings*

Olive oil spray

1 turnip

4 parsnips

2 beets

8 baby carrots

1 rutabaga

1 tablespoon extra-virgin olive oil

Preheat the oven to 450°F. Coat a baking pan with a few spritzes of olive oil. Scrub the vegetables; peel if desired. Cut all the veggies into approximately 1-inch chunks. Place the olive oil in zipper-type plastic bag and add the veggies, shaking to evenly coat with oil. Arrange the veggies in the pan. Roast for 25 to 30 minutes, turning occasionally, or until the veggies are nicely browned. *Winter and late Autumn Fat Flush*

Orange-Scented Roasted Brussels Sprouts

This dish will make some of you wonder why you've been avoiding Brussels sprouts for so long. *Makes about four 1-cup servings*

Olive oil spray

1 pound Brussels sprouts, tough outer
    leaves removed

4 teaspoons macadamia nut oil

1 tablespoon grated orange zest

1 teaspoon dried basil

Preheat the oven to 425°F. In a medium-size bowl, toss the Brussels sprouts with the remaining ingredients. Coat a rimmed baking sheet or casserole dish with a few spritzes of olive oil. Place the Brussels sprouts in a single layer on the baking sheet. Roast for 15 to 20 minutes, or until browned and tender.

Notes from the Fat Flush Kitchen

Roasting the Brussels sprouts brings out their unique and subtle flavor. Look for young Brussels sprouts, found especially at farmers' markets. *Winter and late Autumn Fat Flush*

Sumpdtuous Side Salads

Artichoke and Hearts of Palm Salad

Ideal for springtime eating and gentle cleansing. *Makes 4 servings (Each serving = 1 tablespoon flaxseed oil)*

1 (14-ounce) can artichoke hearts, rinsed
    and drained

1 (14-ounce) can hearts of palm, rinsed
    and drained

1 clove garlic, minced

¼ cup flaxseed oil

2 tablespoons freshly squeezed lemon juice

1 tablespoon apple cider vinegar

1 cup minced fresh parsley

Cayenne

In a medium-size bowl; toss all the ingredients together. Refrigerate for 1 hour prior to serving to allow the flavors to blend. *All seasons*

Beet and Fresh Herbs Salad with Macadamia Nut Oil Vinaigrette

Macadamia nut oil lends an unexpected burst of flavor to this delicious beet salad that is all dressed up with fresh herbs and goat cheese. *Makes 4 servings*

Vinaigrette

    ¼ cup macadamia nut oil

1 tablespoon apple cider vinegar

1 tablespoon freshly squeezed lime juice

6 macadamia nuts, chopped

Pinch of salt (optional)

Salad

8 small beets

4 cups mixed salad greens (baby spinach, endive, watercress, Bibb lettuce)

½ cup fresh parsley leaves, chopped

½ cup fresh marjoram leaves, chopped

½ cup fresh basil leaves, chopped

½ cup mint leaves, chopped finely

4 ounces goat cheese, crumbled

6 macadamia nuts, chopped

Prepare the Vinaigrette

Combine all the ingredients in a jar with a tight-fitting lid; shake well.

Prepare the Salad

Steam the beets; drain, peel, and cut into cubes. On each plate, arrange equal amounts of salad greens, herbs, and beets. Top with equal amounts of goat cheese and chopped macadamia nuts. Drizzle with the vinaigrette.

Notes from the Fat Flush Kitchen

Look for tiny young beets (often available at farmers' markets) as they are more tender. To steam beets, place just enough water in a saucepan so not to touch the steamer. Place the beets in a single layer inside the steamer. Cover; bring the water to a gentle boil. Steam for about 15 minutes; or until fork-tender. Vary the herbs according to your taste and what is available locally. *Winter and late Autumn Fat Flush*

Bitter Greens Salad with Citrus-Infused Vinaigrette

Dandelion greens are just right for springtime eating or a summer salad spectacular like this, with shredded mozzarella and toasted almonds. *Makes 4 servings*

Vinaigrette

2 tablespoons freshly squeezed orange juice

2 tablespoons freshly squeezed lime juice

1 teaspoon orange zest

1 teaspoon lime zest

2 teaspoons apple cider vinegar

2 teaspoons Dijon mustard

2 teaspoons Flora-Key

¼ cup olive oil

Salad

1 small bunch dandelion greens

1 small head endive

1 small head watercress

1 small head radicchio

½ red onion, cut into thin slices

4 ounces mozzarella, shredded

¼ cup dried tart cherries

½ cup almonds, toasted

Prepare the Vinaigrette
Combine all the vinaigrette ingredients except the oil in a blender or food
processor. Slowly add the oil, blending until the vinaigrette is thickened.
Prepare the Salad
Combine all the salad ingredients in a large bowl; toss with the vinaigrette.
Feasts and festivities

SASSY SOUPS
    Survival Soup
    Curried Delicata Squash Bisque
    Beet Borscht

Survival Soup

My full-bodied soup is a meal-in-one that Fat Flushers have come to rely on.—
Linda S., Naples, Florida. *Makes about ten 2-cup servings*

Olive oil spray
2 pounds lean ground beef or turkey
2 onions, chopped coarsely
2 bell peppers, seeded and chopped
    coarsely
1 pound mushrooms, any variety,
    chopped coarsely
3 cloves garlic, chopped
2 medium-size eggplant, peeled and
    cubed
1 (28-ounce) can whole tomatoes,

    chopped coarsely
1 (28-ounce) can crushed tomatoes
1 (28-ounce) can tomato puree
1 strip kombu
32 ounces (1 quart) beef broth
Cayenne
2 tablespoons ground cumin
½ bunch fresh cilantro, chopped
½ bunch fresh parsley, chopped

Lightly coat the bottom of a stockpot with a few spritzes of olive oil; heat over
medium-high heat. Sauté the beef for about 5 minutes, or until no pink remains;
drain well; set aside. Sauté the onion, peppers, mushrooms, garlic, and eggplant
for about 5 minutes, or until the veggies are softened. Add the tomatoes, tomato
puree, kombu, broth, and reserved meat; cover and simmer for 15 to 20 minutes.
Stir in the cayenne to taste, cumin, cilantro, and parsley. Cook for about 10
minutes longer to blend the flavors. Remove the kombu.

Notes from the Fat Flush Kitchen
This soup is adaptable to any combination of veggies you like. Don't shy away from
herbs and spices! For a Middle Eastern taste, add some coriander. In Winter and
Spring Fat Flush, try an Italian twist by adding oregano and basil. For Autumn,

use veggie broth instead of the beef broth and omit the ground beef or turkey. You may also add 2 pounds of firm tofu, cut into cubes. *Winter, Spring and Summer*

Curried Delicata Squash Bisque

This is an excellent soup for a chilly autumn or winter evening. Delicata squash is very tender and cooks more quickly than other winter squashes. The spices are very warming. The apple cider vinegar adds a tartness that brings out the apples.—Debbie B., Chicago, Illinois. *Makes about six 1-cup servings*

3 pounds Delicata squash (or other
   winter squash), peeled and seeded, cut
   in chunks
2 apples, peeled and cored
2 leeks, washed well and trimmed

1 teaspoon ground ginger
1 teaspoon ground coriander
½ teaspoon ground cumin
⅓ cup apple cider vinegar
2 cups vegetable broth

Steam the squash, apples, and leeks for about 8 minutes, or until tender. In a food processor, chop the mixture lightly, leaving some chunks. Place the mixture in a soup pot; simmer over medium-low heat for about 20 minutes. Stir in the spices, apple cider vinegar, and veggie broth. Simmer for about 5 minutes longer. Winter, Spring, and late Autumn Fat Flush

Beet Borscht

This recipe was adapted from an old family favorite, using whatever seasonal veggies are available. The addition of stewed beef or chicken would bump it up to a complete meal in a bowl!—Nina M., Chemainus, British Columbia. *Makes about twelve 2-cup servings*

8 medium-size red beets with stalks and
   greens
Cold water
8 cups vegetable broth
2 medium-size onions, chopped
½ small red cabbage, chopped
½ small green cabbage, chopped
3 medium-size carrots, peeled and
   chopped

3 stalks celery, chopped
3 cloves garlic, chopped
1 jalapeño, seeded and diced
1 small bunch kale (about ½ pound),
   stalks removed
1 (28-ounce) can diced tomatoes
3 tablespoons apple cider vinegar
Fresh dill sprigs

Remove the stalks and greens from the beets; coarsely chop and reserve. In a large soup pot, cover the beets with cold water; bring to a boil; boil the beets for 2 minutes; rinse in a strainer under cold water. Peel and chop the beets; return to the soup pot. Add the broth, onions, cabbage, carrots, celery, garlic, and jalapeño. Bring to a boil; simmer for about 30 minutes, or until the veggies are almost tender. Add the beet stalks and greens, kale, tomatoes, and apple cider vinegar. Simmer until the kale is tender, 20 to 30 minutes. If desired, puree one-third to half of the soup in a food processor or with a handheld blender. Garnish with the dill sprigs. Serve hot or chilled.

Notes from the Fat Flush Kitchen
For a more delicate flavor and gorgeous amber hue, try using golden beets. If you like, you may top each serving with a dollop of sour cream. This soup will feed a crowd! You may want to consider halving the recipe or freezing leftovers for a future use. *Winter and late Autumn Fat Flush*

FLAVORFUL FAVORITES: SEASONINGS, CONDIMENTS, AND SALAD DRESSINGS

Garam Masala   E-Z Fat Flush Vinaigrette
Fat Flush Seasoning   Amazing Caesar Dressing
E-Z Classic Mayo   Herbal Dijon Vinaigrette
Roasted Red Pepper Sauce   Mediterranean Vinaigrette
Fresh Cranberry Chutney   Sesame Vinaigrette

Garam Masala

My garam masala is a variation of a traditional blend. It adds unexpected flavor to everything from morning eggs to baked apples as well as stir-fries.—Charli S., Beverly, Washington. *Makes about ¼ cup plus 2 tablespoons*

4 teaspoons ground cloves   *4 teaspoons ground cumin*
2 tablespoons ground cinnamon   *4 teaspoons ground coriander*

Combine all the ingredients. Place in a covered container or shaker bottle. Store the garam masala at room temperature away from the stove. *All seasons*

Fat Flush Seasoning

Fat Flush Seasoning is so versatile! Try it on fish, seafood, beef, poultry, and lamb dishes—and that's just for starters! Even your morning eggs will wake up with just a sprinkle. *Makes approximately ½ cup*

2 tablespoons onion powder	1 teaspoon minced lemon zest
2 tablespoons garlic powder	¼ teaspoon cayenne
2 teaspoons ground coriander	¼ cup ground cumin
¼ cup dried parsley	½ packet Stevia Plus

Combine all the ingredients. Place in a covered container or shaker bottle. Store the seasoning at room temperature away from the stove. *All seasons*

E-Z Classic Mayo

Once you try this homemade "classic" mayo, I think you'll agree it tastes so much better than those store-bought brands with unwholesome ingredients. *Makes about 2 cups or sixteen 2-tablespoon servings (Each serving = 1 tablespoon flaxseed oil)*

1 clove garlic	2 tablespoons apple cider vinegar
Pinch of dry mustard	Cayenne
2 large egg yolks	1 cup flaxseed oil
2 tablespoons freshly squeezed lemon juice	

In a food processor or blender, blend all the ingredients except the oil. Drizzle in the oil until the mixture thickens into mayonnaise. Store the mayonnaise in a covered container in the refrigerator.

Notes from the Fat Flush Kitchen

For Fresh Herbed Mayonnaise: Mix in ½ cup minced fresh green herbs (dill, cilantro, parsley, etc.). Thin with a few drops of filtered water, if desired. For Winter Fat Flush, try macadamia nut or extra-virgin olive oil which, unlike flaxseed oil, can be used in cooking and heated dishes. *All seasons*

Roasted Red Pepper Sauce

This vibrant sauce dresses up everything from main dishes to sides. I use it as a salad dressing! *Makes about 1 cup or four ¼-cup servings (Each serving = 1 tablespoon flaxseed oil)*

2 red bell peppers, seeded, quartered,
  and roasted
2 cloves garlic, minced
¼ cup flaxseed oil

2 teaspoons chopped fresh parsley
2 teaspoons freshly squeezed lemon or
  lime juice
½ teaspoon dry mustard

Blend all the ingredients until smooth. Store the sauce in a covered container in the refrigerator.

Notes from the Fat Flush Kitchen

Keep in mind this sauce cannot be heated as it contains flaxseed oil, which is fragile. However, you can serve it as a dip or spooned over hot foods such as eggs, veggies, chicken, beef, seafood, and so on.

To roast a pepper: Place cut side down on a pan. Roast at 450°F until the pepper is blackened (about 10 minutes). Remove from the oven. When cool enough to handle, remove the blackened skin and discard. *All seasons*

Fresh Cranberry Chutney

Freshen up your holiday turkey and chicken dishes with this ruby-colored chutney. *Makes about eight 1-cup servings*

2 cups apple, peeled, cored, and chopped
4 cups fresh or frozen cranberries
¼ cup chopped onion
2 stalks celery, chopped
1 red bell pepper, seeded and chopped
½ cup apple cider vinegar

1 tablespoon grated fresh ginger, or 1
  teaspoon ground
1 teaspoon ground cinnamon
Zest from 1 orange
1 tablespoon Flora-Key

Combine all the ingredients except Flora-Key in a 2-quart saucepan. Simmer for 20 to 25 minutes, or until all veggies and fruits are tender, stirring often. Let cool; stir in the Flora-Key. Store the chutney in a covered container in the refrigerator until serving.

Notes from the Fat Flush Kitchen

For feasts and festivities, you may add a tablespoon of honey for extra sweetness. *All seasons*

E-Z Fat Flush Vinaigrette

This basic vinaigrette whips up in just minutes! *Makes about ½ cup (four 2-tablespoon servings) (Each serving = 1 tablespoon oil)*

¼ cup flaxseed oil or lemon-flavored fish oil

2 tablespoons apple cider vinegar

2 tablespoons freshly squeezed lemon or lime juice

1 clove garlic

1 tablespoon chopped fresh parsley

1 tablespoon chopped fresh cilantro

Pinch of dry mustard

Cayenne

Place all the ingredients in a glass container with a lid; shake well. Store the vinaigrette in the refrigerator.

Notes from the Fat Flush Kitchen

Just a friendly reminder—flaxseed oil is fragile, so it cannot be used in dishes that require heating. In Winter Fat Flush, try replacing the flaxseed oil with extra-virgin olive oil, coconut oil, or macadamia nut oil. *All seasons*

Amazing Caesar Dressing

It's quite delicious with any greens such as baby spinach, bitter lettuces, mild Bibb, and even arugula and radicchio. *Makes about 1 cup (eight 2-tablespoon servings) (Each serving = 1 tablespoon oil)*

1 large egg, raw or coddled

Grated zest from 1 lemon

Juice from 1 small lemon

1 to 2 garlic cloves

¼ to ½ teaspoon dry mustard

Pinch of salt (optional)

2 tablespoons apple cider vinegar

½ cup flaxseed oil

Place all ingredients except the flaxseed oil in blender or food processor. Drizzle in the flaxseed oil and blend until thickened and smooth. Store the dressing in the refrigerator. *All seasons*

Herbal Dijon Vinaigrette

This vinaigrette is so easy and delicious, you'll use it all the time and start taking it to restaurants. *Makes about 1 cup (eight 2-tablespoon servings) (Each serving = 1 tablespoon oil)*

½ cup apple cider vinegar
½ cup flaxseed oil or lemon-flavored
   fish oil
2 cloves garlic, crushed

1 teaspoon Dijon mustard, or to taste
1 teaspoon minced fresh parsley
1 teaspoon minced fresh dill
1 teaspoon minced green onions

Place all ingredients in a glass container with a lid; shake well. Store the vinaigrette in the refrigerator.

Notes from the Fat Flush Kitchen

In Autumn Fat Flush, use flaxseed oil instead of fish oil. In Summer Fat Flush use ¼ teaspoon of dry mustard instead of Dijon mustard. *Winter and Spring Fat Flush*

Mediterranean Vinaigrette

This traditional Fat Flush dressing is a lovely base for lots of additional seasonings such as shallots, chives, fresh basil, and capers (Winter Fat Flush). *Makes about ten 2-tablespoon servings (Each serving = about 1 tablespoon oil)*

½ cup flaxseed oil
¼ cup apple cider vinegar
¼ cup freshly squeezed lemon juice
¼ cup roasted red peppers

1½ teaspoons Dijon mustard
1 clove garlic
8 black olives
Cayenne

Place all the ingredients in a blender. Blend until the peppers and olives are finely minced. Store the vinaigrette in the refrigerator. *Winter, Spring, and mid-Autumn Fat Flush*

Sesame Vinaigrette

Sesame Vinaigrette really shines when drizzled on steamed veggies. Its distinct, nutty taste is enhanced by mustard and Seaweed Gomasio seasoning. *Makes about 1 cup (eight 2-tablespoon servings) (Each serving = 1 tablespoon oil)*

½ cup toasted sesame oil
¼ cup apple cider vinegar
¼ cup freshly squeezed lime juice

¼ teaspoon dry mustard
2 teaspoons Seaweed Gomasio

Place all the ingredients in a glass container with a lid; shake well. Store the vinaigrette in the refrigerator. *Winter and late Autumn Fat Flush*

NOT-TOO-SWEET TREATS

Ginger Peach Sorbet

Fruit Kebabs with Wild Berry Coulis

Sweetie Po' Puffs

Black 'n' White Yogurt Parfait

Maple-Infused Pears

Summer Fruit Crumble

Hungarian Almond Torte

Favorite Pumpkin Pie

Tart Cherry Kanten

Chocolate Bliss Fondue

Ginger Peach Sorbet

In this dessert, adapted from a recipe from one of my Fat Flushers, the hot and pungent qualities of ginger deliciously contrast with the cooling peach sorbet. *Makes about four cups or four 1-cup servings*

20 frozen peach sections (or equivalent of 4 peaches)

Juice of 1 lemon

Juice of 1 lime

Grated zest of 1 lemon half

Grated zest of 1 lime half

1½ teaspoons grated fresh ginger

4 teaspoons Flora-Key

Pinch of cayenne

Using a blender or food processor, blend all the ingredients until slushy. Serve immediately as a delicious soft sorbet or freeze, thawing about 15 minutes before serving. *All seasons*

Fruit Kebabs with Wild Berry Coulis

What a great way to take advantage of the fruits of the season! *Makes 4 servings*

Wild Berry Coulis

1 cup frozen mixed berries

Kebabs

1 apple

1 pear

1 peach

1 cup blackberries

Prepare the Wild Berry Coulis

Let the frozen mixed berries stand at room temperature just until semisoft. Puree in a blender or food processor until almost smooth with small berry chunks remaining.

Prepare the Kebabs
Core the apple and pear and cut into chunks. Thread the apple and pear pieces and the berries alternatively on four wooden skewers. Drizzle each kebab with 1 tablespoon of Wild Berry Coulis.

Notes from the Fat Flush Kitchen
Let your little ones wear the chef's hat by letting them help to put together this colorful and nutritious snack. Look for skewers with blunt ends, to protect tiny hands. *All seasons*

Sweetie Po' Puffs

Sweet veggies make superb snacks...no sugar and lots of fiber, too! I love the orange zest in this cookie. And it's so portable...a great power snack for the road!—Sarah W., Yarmouth, Maine
Makes 4 servings

16 ounces sweet potato, cooked and   *Zest from ½ orange*
    chilled   *1 orange, peeled and seeded*
2 large eggs   *½ teaspoon ground ginger*
2 servings Fat Flush Vanilla Whey   *1 teaspoon ground cinnamon*
    Protein   *¼ cup chia seeds*

Preheat the oven to 350°F. Line a baking sheet with parchment paper. Place all the ingredients in a blender or food processor and mix until smooth, adding drizzles of water if the mixture is too thick. (Do not thin the batter more than necessary—the mixture should remain thick.) Using a ¼-cup measure, form into sixteen mounds on the prepared baking sheet. Flatten with a spatula into circles. Bake for 25 to 30 minutes, until the cookies are puffed, golden, and firm. Remove from the oven and let cool thoroughly before removing from the pan. Refrigerate in a loosely covered container, separating layers with waxed paper.

Notes from the Fat Flush Kitchen
Try replacing the orange and the orange zest with a chopped, peeled apple. In Winter Fat Flush, cardamom provides a touch of exotic flavor. These soft cookies look lovely on a buffet table with a bowl of Wild Berry Coulis (page 239) for dipping. *Winter, Spring, and late Autumn Fat Flush*

Black 'n' White Yogurt Parfait

A tease of vanilla and chocolate flavors swirled together with a bit of crunch...the perfect craving buster! *Makes 1 serving*

1 cup plain yogurt
½ serving Fat Flush Vanilla Whey
   Protein
½ serving Fat Flush Chocolate Whey
   Protein

1 tablespoon chia seeds
⅛ teaspoon ground cinnamon
1 teaspoon Flora-Key

Mix ½ cup of the yogurt with the vanilla whey. Mix the remaining yogurt with the chocolate whey. Set aside. Mix the chia seeds with the cinnamon and Flora-Key. In a glass or parfait dish, alternate layers of the vanilla yogurt mixture, chia seed mixture, and chocolate yogurt mixture, repeating as needed. *Winter and Autumn Fat Flush*

Maple-Infused Pears

Go ahead and indulge. This elegant and no-fuss dessert provides a sweet and warming touch to dinner. *Makes 4 servings*

Pears
   Olive oil spray
   4 medium-firm pears, cored and
   quartered
   ¼ cup pure maple syrup
   2 tablespoons chopped walnuts

Cacao-Cinnamon Sprinkle
   2 tablespoons cacao powder
   4 teaspoons Flora-Key
   ¼ teaspoon ground cinnamon

Prepare the Pears
Preheat the oven to 350°F. Lightly coat an 8-inch square baking dish with a few spritzes of olive oil; arrange the pears in the dish. Drizzle the maple syrup over the pears. Scatter the walnuts over the pears. Bake until the pears are soft but not mushy, approximately 20 minutes, basting after 10 minutes. Let cool slightly. Dust with half of the Cacao-Cinnamon Sprinkle (reserve rest for another use).
Prepare the Cacao-Cinnamon Sprinkle
In a small bowl or shaker bottle, mix together all the ingredients. *Feasts and festivities*

Summer Fruit Crumble

What better way to capture the essence of summer than with peaches and fresh berries. *Makes 8 servings*

Olive oil spray

Filling
  4 peaches or nectarines, cut into slices
  ¼ cup raspberries
  ¼ cup blackberries
  1 tablespoon oat flour
  1 packet Stevia Plus
  2 tablespoons freshly squeezed lemon juice
  ¼ cup toasted chopped almonds

Crust
  ⅓ cup oat flour
  1 serving Fat Flush Vanilla Whey Protein
  3 packets Stevia Plus
  ½ teaspoon ground cinnamon
  2 tablespoons unsalted butter, chilled, cut into bits
  ½ cup rolled oats, soaked in ½ cup water until softened, about 10 minutes

Preheat the oven to 375°F. Lightly coat an 8-inch square baking pan with a few spritzes of olive oil.

Prepare the Filling

In a medium-size bowl, combine the fruit. In a small bowl, combine the oat flour and Stevia Plus, then add the lemon juice, stirring until the Stevia Plus has dissolved. Toss the lemon juice mixture with the fruit and the almonds. Pour the filling into the baking pan.

Prepare the Crust

In a medium-size bowl, stir together the oat flour, whey protein, Stevia Plus, and cinnamon. With two knives or a pastry blender, cut in the butter until pea-size lumps form. Stir in the softened oats, forming a thick paste. (Stir in a few drops of water if the oat mixture is too thick.) Carefully spread the crust over the filling. Bake for 40 to 45 minutes, or until the filling is bubbly and the crust is browned and crispy. *Feasts and festivities*

Hungarian Almond Torte

Incredibly light, this torte makes a lovely dessert for year-round celebrations. *Makes 12 servings (one 10-inch cake)*

Olive oil spray
6 large or 7 medium-size eggs, separated
½ teaspoon cream of tartar
2 teaspoons almond extract
Juice and zest of 1 lemon

3 tablespoons honey
1½ cups almond meal
Cacao-Cinnamon Sprinkle (page 241)
⅓ cup chopped almonds, toasted

Preheat the oven to 350°F. Line the bottom of a 10-inch tube-shaped springform or tube pan with parchment paper. Lightly coat the parchment paper and sides of the pan with a few spritzes of olive oil. In a large mixing bowl, beat the egg whites with the cream of tartar until stiff but not dry. In a medium-size bowl, beat the egg yolks with the almond extract, lemon juice and zest, honey, and almond meal. Gently fold into the egg white mixture. Carefully pour the batter into the pan. Bake for 25 to 30 minutes, or until a knife inserted into the center comes out clean. Let cool for 5 minutes. Run a knife around the sides of the pan; carefully transfer the cake to a cooling rack. Let cool for 10 minutes. Transfer the cake to a serving plate. Dust the top of the torte with Cacao-Cinnamon Sprinkle and top with chopped almonds.

Notes from the Fat Flush Kitchen

This torte would look beautiful surrounded by a garland of fresh berries. *Feasts and festivities*

Favorite Pumpkin Pie

This pumpkin pie is mighty high in protein so I would eat it for breakfast on those special occasions!—Jenny M., St. Helens, Oregon. *Makes 8 servings (one 9-inch pie)*

Crust
  1¼ cups spelt flour
  Pinch of salt
  1 packet Stevia Plus
  3 tablespoons Fat Flush Vanilla
  Whey Protein mixed with 3
  tablespoons water
  ¼ cup macadamia nut oil

Filling
  1 (15-ounce) can unsweetened solid
  pumpkin
  ¼ cup plus 2 tablespoons Fat Flush
  Vanilla Whey Protein blended with
  ½ cup water
  1 teaspoon each ground cinnamon
  and nutmeg

Filling (continued)
    ½ teaspoon ground ginger
    ¼ teaspoon ground cloves
    1 teaspoon salt

3 packets Stevia Plus
3 tablespoons honey
2 large eggs, beaten lightly

Preheat the oven to 425°F.

Prepare the Crust

In a medium-size bowl, stir together the spelt flour, salt, and Stevia Plus. In a small bowl, stir together the whey mixture and oil. Add the wet ingredients to the dry, mixing well. Form the crust mixture into a ball; press onto the bottom of a 9-inch pie plate and 1 inch up the sides.

Prepare the Filling

In a large bowl, blend together the pumpkin, 2 tablespoons of the whey mixture, the spices, and the salt. Add the remaining filling ingredients. Mix gently just until all the ingredients are thoroughly combined. Pour the filling into the pie crust. Bake for 15 minutes; lower the heat to 350°F and bake for an additional 40 minutes, or until a knife inserted into the center comes out clean. Check the pie after about 25 minutes. If the outside is getting too brown, cover the edges with foil. *Feasts and festivities*

Tart Cherry Kanten

Dessert is just a bowl of cherries! *Makes four ¾-cup servings*

2 cups tart cherry juice
¼ cup agar flakes
⅛ teaspoon ground cinnamon
⅛ teaspoon ground cloves

2 tablespoons chopped pecans
½ cup unsweetened dried tart cherries
4 teaspoons Flora-Key (optional)

In a small saucepan, stir together cherry juice and agar flakes; let stand for 10 minutes. Stir in the spices, pecans, and cherries; bring to a boil over low heat, stirring occasionally. Continue to boil for 30 seconds; remove from the heat. Pour into four parfait glasses. Let cool for about 15 minutes. Refrigerate for about an hour until firm. Before serving, sprinkle each cup with 1 teaspoon Flora-Key, if desired.

Notes from the Fat Flush Kitchen

Kanten is a Japanese gelled dish. It is made from agar, which is a gel-like substance found in seaweed. Kanten dishes can be enjoyed as a dessert or a savory side dish made with vegetables. *Feasts and festivities*

Chocolate Bliss Fondue

The name says it all. For those special occasions, a little bit of chocolate goes a long way. *Makes 4 servings*

4 ounces unsweetened dark chocolate,
   chopped coarsely
1 tablespoon unsalted butter

4 teaspoons honey
4 cups fresh fruit (strawberries, banana
   chunks, orange wedges, kiwi, etc.)

In the top of a double boiler, over simmering water, melt the chocolate, butter, and honey, stirring occasionally. Remove from the heat; let cool slightly. Skewer the fruit on toothpicks and dip into the chocolate.

Notes from the Fat Flush Kitchen
If you don't have a double boiler, two pots that fit on top of each other will do just fine. *Feasts and festivities*

SNACK ATTACK!

Spinach "Flatbread"
Fabulous Chia Crax
Chunky Artichoke Dip
Roasted Eggplant Spread
Lemony Tapenade

Just Vegg 'n-Out Munchies
Crunchy Chickpeas
Chickpea Tahini Pâté
Ginger-Honey Yogurt Dip

Spinach "Flatbread"

This is a simple, no-fail recipe. You don't really have to measure the ingredients, and the variations are endless! It freezes beautifully and grills or toasts well, too.—Rachel T., Canada
Makes 1 to 2 servings

1 (10-ounce) package frozen chopped
   spinach, thawed and drained
2 large eggs

2 large egg whites
½ teaspoon minced garlic
¼ cup chopped onions

Preheat the oven to 400°F. In a mixing bowl, stir together all the ingredients. Line a baking sheet with parchment paper; pour the mixture evenly onto the pan. Bake for 15 minutes. Holding the ends of the parchment paper, pick up the flatbread and lay on a cooling rack or towel. Cut into sandwich or wrap-size pieces and load with your favorite toppings.

Notes from the Fat Flush Kitchen

Try adding ¼ cup each chopped red and orange bell peppers to provide a colorful contrast to the bright green spinach. One-quarter cup each of chopped artichokes or water chestnuts are delicious additions as well. In Winter and Spring Fat Flush, sprinkle with a pinch of basil and oregano for an Italian twist. This "flatbread" has so many functions…cut into wedges and top with your favorite veggies or spreads. Or cut it into squares, fill with tuna or egg salad, and it becomes a wrap. Its uses are only limited by your creativity! *All seasons*

Fabulous Chia Crax

The perfect cracker that you can bring with you to satisfy that midmorning or midafternoon craving. *Makes 16 servings (Each cracker = about 1 tablespoon chia seeds)*

Chia Gel
  ⅓ cup chia seeds
  2 cups water

Crackers
  ¾ cup chia seeds

2 packets Stevia Plus
1 tablespoon ground cinnamon
½ teaspoon ground ginger
½ cup Chia Gel (see left column)

Prepare the Chia Gel

In a container with a lid, combine the chia seeds and water. Cover; shake for 45 seconds. Let the mixture rest for 1 minute; shake again. Let the mixture rest for 15 minutes before using. Store leftover Chia Gel in the refrigerator for up to 2 weeks.

Prepare the Crackers

Preheat the oven to 275°F. In a medium-size bowl, combine the chia seeds, Stevia Plus, and spices. Add the Chia Gel, stirring until well mixed and the seeds start to form a ball (about 5 minutes). Line a baking sheet with parchment paper. Spoon the chia seed mixture onto the baking sheet. Cover with another sheet of parchment paper. Using a glass or rolling pin, roll the mixture flat and out to the sides of the baking sheet. When the mixture is evenly distributed, remove and discard the top parchment paper. Score the dough lightly into sixteen crackers, using a pizza cutter or fork. Bake for 45 minutes to 1 hour, or until the crackers pull away from the parchment paper and separate easily. Store the crackers in an airtight container at room temperature.

Notes from the Fat Flush Kitchen

Prefer savory over sweet? Simply replace the cinnamon, ginger, and Stevia Plus with such flavorings as fennel, onion, or garlic powder, cayenne, cumin, or dill. In Spring Fat Flush, try basil or oregano. In Winter Fat Flush, what about cardamom or nutmeg? Get creative using Chia Gel! Stir it into such foods as dips, salad dressings, sauces, drinks, and oatmeal for an added nutritional boost. Chia Gel also acts as a natural thickener and fat replacer without affecting flavor. *All seasons*

Chunky Artichoke Dip

Artichokes and water chestnuts play the starring role in this delicious dip. Perfect for hors d'oeuvres to bring to potlucks, parties, and picnics when you want to show off. *Makes about 2½ cups, or five ½-cup servings*

1 (14-ounce) can artichoke hearts, drained and chopped
1 (7-ounce) can water chestnuts, drained and chopped
¼ cup seeded and diced red bell pepper

½ cup E-Z Classic Mayo (page 235)
1 tablespoon freshly squeezed lemon juice
¼ cup chopped fresh parsley
Cayenne

In medium-size bowl, stir together all the ingredients; chill. Store the dip in a covered container in the refrigerator. *All seasons*

Roasted Eggplant Spread

An easy way to bring out the meaty, full-bodied texture and smoky taste of eggplant. *Makes about 2 cups, or four ½-cup servings*

Olive oil spray
1 large eggplant, roasted
½ cup minced fresh cilantro
½ cup minced fresh parsley
¼ cup seeded and chopped red and/or orange bell pepper

1 clove garlic, minced
2 tablespoons freshly squeezed lime juice
1 teaspoon ground cumin
Cayenne
Sliced green onions, for garnish

Into a medium-size bowl, scrape the flesh of the roasted eggplant; mash coarsely. Stir in the remaining ingredients except the green onions. Top with the sliced green onions. Chill for about 30 minutes to allow the flavors to blend. Serve with your favorite veggie dippers.

Notes from the Fat Flush Kitchen

To roast an eggplant: Preheat the oven to 450F. Lightly coat a rimmed baking pan with a few spritzes of olive oil. Remove the stem from the eggplant and cut in half lengthwise. Place flesh side down on the baking pan. Roast for about 15 minutes, or until the skin becomes darkened and begins to collapse. The flesh should be very soft. Let cool. *All seasons*

Lemony Tapenade

Enjoy this lovely tapenade with fresh veggie dippers or as a topping for chicken and fish year round. *Makes about 1 cup or four ¼-cup servings*

1 cup black olives	*1 to 2 garlic cloves, minced*
4 teaspoons flaxseed oil	*Pinch of cayenne*
1 tablespoon freshly squeezed lemon juice	

In a blender or food processor, process all the ingredients until chunky. Store the tapenade in a covered container in the refrigerator. *All seasons*

Just Vegg'n-Out Munchies

How do I love veggies? Let me count the ways. ...*Makes about four 2-cup servings*

Veggies	*1 cup chopped fresh fennel*
1 cup broccoli or cauliflower florets	*1 cup chopped fresh parsley*
1 red bell pepper (or any color), seeded and cut into chunks	*1 cup chopped fresh cilantro*
8 baby carrots, sliced	*Marinade*
4 stalks celery, chopped	*¼ cup flaxseed oil*
2 cups shredded green or red cabbage	*½ cup apple cider vinegar*
¼ cup black olives, sliced	*1 tablespoon Seaweed Gomasio*

Prepare the Veggies
In a large, shallow, nonmetal container (with a lid if possible), combine the veggies and herbs.
Prepare the Marinade
In a small bowl, stir together the oil, vinegar, and Seaweed Gomasio. Pour the oil and vinegar mixture over the vegetables. Cover; shake well. Refrigerate the veggies for several hours or overnight, shaking the container occasionally to evenly distribute the marinade. *All seasons*

Crunchy Chickpeas

No need to reach for potato chips when you can grab these spiced-up chickpeas instead. *Makes about 2 cups or four ½-cup servings*

Olive oil spray
1 (14-ounce) can chickpeas (garbanzo beans), rinsed and drained
⅛ teaspoon garlic powder (or other spices as desired)

⅛ teaspoon onion powder (or other spices as desired)
Cayenne

Preheat the oven to 325°F. Lightly coat a rimmed baking sheet with spritzes of olive oil. In a small bowl, toss the chickpeas with a few spritzes of olive oil and spices. Spread out the chickpeas on the baking sheet. Roast, shaking the pan about every 15 minutes, until the chickpeas are browned and crunchy, about 30 minutes. Let cool before serving. Store the chickpeas in a covered container at room temperature.

Notes from the Fat Flush Kitchen

Sweet tooth? Try replacing the garlic and onion powder with ground cinnamon and ginger. *Mid-Winter and Autumn Fat Flush*

Chickpea Tahini Pâté

With lots of antioxidant power from spices, as a snack or main meal, this Mideast pâté is satisfying and fiber-rich. *Makes about 2 cups or four ½-cup servings*

1 (14-ounce) can chickpeas (garbanzos); reserve liquid
¼ cup diced onion
2 tablespoons chopped fresh parsley
2 tablespoons chopped fresh cilantro
1 clove garlic, minced

½ teaspoon ground cumin
2 tablespoons sesame seed butter (tahini)
1 teaspoon Seaweed Gomasio
Cayenne
3 tablespoons freshly squeezed lemon juice

In a blender or food processor, blend all the ingredients until the desired consistency is reached. If too thick, add a few drops of the reserved liquid. *Mid-Winter and Autumn Fat Flush*

Ginger-Honey Yogurt Dip

Sweet and warming, this dip goes well with Roasted Root Veggies (page 229) or drizzled over a warm baked apple. *Makes about four ½-cup servings*

2 cups plain yogurt
1 tablespoon honey
1 teaspoon grated fresh ginger

In a medium-size bowl, blend all the ingredients together. Store the dip in a covered container in the refrigerator.

Notes from the Fat Flush Kitchen

For an especially thick and creamy texture, try plain Greek yogurt. *Feasts and festivities*

APPENDIX: THE 5-DAY HOT METABOLISM BOOSTER: BREAKING WEIGHT-LOSS PLATEAUS

Doing the same thing over and over again but expecting different results is the definition of insanity.

—*Albert Einstein*

SO, YOU'RE SEVERAL MONTHS into one of the seasonal Fat Flush programs and the scale is stuck. Your resolve is beginning to wane, you're having trouble sticking to the plan, and you are frustrated that the scale is not moving southward as quickly and effortlessly as it once did. Or maybe you celebrated a little too much during the holidays or you just got back from a "fattening" vacation. Don't worry. In five days, you will right back on track where you left off. You may even be a good five to ten pounds lighter.

Everyone hits a weight-loss plateau at some point and needs a slump-busting plan to get those pounds moving again. (A plateau is defined as a three-week period when the scale doesn't budge.) Maybe there's a wedding coming up or your twentieth high school reunion and you need to lose weight right away. Or maybe you have a little black dress or certain tux hanging in your closet that you plan to wear next weekend and you need an "emergency" way to lose your tummy in a hurry. Whatever your reason, this plan is going to be your new Fat Flush BF.

ENTER THE 5-DAY HOT METABOLISM BOOSTER

I wanted to help people recoup their "skinny" metabolisms and break their weight-loss plateaus by following a plan that would be amazingly satisfying and effective. The plan, originally created for a national women's magazine in December 2004, has since morphed from a three-day regimen into a really "hot" five-day weight-loss buster—one that is guaranteed to work more rapidly than even the popular Cabbage Soup Diet. The plan has enjoyed tremendous success from the members of my online community and remains today one of my most requested diets. Probably the most surprising and gratifying beneficial side effect is that it prevents rebound weight gain so common on most "crash" diets.

WHY YOU'LL GET RESULTS

The centerpiece of the plan is a cocktail called the Hot Metabolism Booster that you will be drinking three times per day: morning, noon, and night. The cocktail, due to its high water content, helps you to get filled up and fuller longer while keeping calories down. As research studies performed at Penn State have shown, individuals who consumed soups twice a day lost twice as much weight as study participants who ate foods with equivalent calories. The souplike consistency of the cocktail allows you to have a larger volume of food, which triggers the stomach's stretch-like receptors to signal the brain, so you stop eating.[1] It's that simple.

HOW YOUR METABOLISM IS KICKED INTO OVERDRIVE

Here is a quick run-down of the plateau-busting ingredients and a simple explanation of how they work. As you take a quick glance, you will see that many of the ingredients are as close as your spice rack. You most likely will already have others on hand because they are Fat Flushing Superfoods.

Tomato or vegetable juice—These high–vitamin C ingredients increase satiety and hunger satisfaction because of their high water content that simulates broth-based meals.

Lemon or lime juice—Studies show that acids enhance the body's ability to emulsify fat.

Parsley—This natural diuretic contains apiole, an organic compound that stimulates the kidneys to rid the body of excess fluids.

Cilantro—A potent detoxifier of such heavy metals as mercury and lead, cilantro, or "Mexican parsley," also helps to relieve bloating.

Green onion—Mineral-rich green onions contain aromatic oils that help break down fatty deposits.

Garlic—Garlic can boost metabolism due to its allicin-rich content that has fat-blasting power.[2]

Cayenne—The compound that gives cayenne its fire, capsaicin, can heat up metabolism as much as 25 percent.

Olive oil—This monounsaturated fatty acid inhibits the buildup of weight in the belly.[3]

Seaweed Gomasio—Iodine-rich Seaweed Gomasio helps to normalize thyroid hormones to blast fat.

Turmeric—A natural anti-inflammatory, turmeric can help thin and decongest bile, so your body can emulsify fat more efficiently.

Flora-Key—The addition of a probiotic will ensure healthy digestion and decrease bloating from yeast overgrowth.

Chia seeds—Fiber-rich chia seeds will help keep blood sugar on an even keel so you are not hungry.

Hot Metabolism Insider Secrets

Here are a few tips and tricks I've gathered from many HMB "junkies":

■ Save time by prepping ingredients ahead of time.

■ Save even more time by mixing up all three cocktails at once. Have one for breakfast, take one to work for an afternoon snack, and keep one ready and waiting in your fridge for after dinner.

■ The meal plans are flexible! Don't care for tilapia? Then choose a fish from the Summer Fat Flushing Superstar Foods. Not a broccoli lover? Any veggie choice from the Summer Fat Flush list will do. Hard-boiled eggs are included for convenience, but any way you prefer eggs is just fine (just no added oil, please). You may also switch lunches and dinners within the same day.

■ Remember, daily weight often fluctuates due to menstrual cycles and even the phases of the moon, so please hide your scale. Weigh yourself on the morning of Day 1 and then be pleasantly surprised the morning of Day 6. Remember, inches count, too, because inch loss equates with fat loss, so don't forget those important before and after measurements. Of course, the best reward of all will be fitting into your favorite "skinny" jeans.

■ If you get hungry, reach for an extra ounce or two of lean protein. You may also enjoy your Cranberry H_2O and snack on any additional Summer Fat Flush–friendly veggies (see page 138). Like the rest of the Fat Flush science, the 5-Day Hot Metabolism Booster continues to define just how on target my plan is—confirming the secrets to success.

OTHER MENU MAINSTAYS

Beverages

Drinking plenty of water between meals is a fundamental principle of Fat Flushing in general. Water not only helps to flush out toxins but also hydrates tissues and revs up metabolism by about 3 percent, according to research studies.

Protein

By filling up on lean protein (eggs, fish, seafood, poultry, and whey) you can raise your metabolism by roughly 25 percent. When the body is deficient in protein, fluid leaks from the vascular spaces into the spaces between the cells and becomes trapped. This results in cellulite, water retention, bloating, and water weight gain. Eating protein stimulates the pancreas to produce glucagon, the hormone that counteracts insulin and mobilizes fat from storage.[4]

Veggies

Green and low-starch vegetables help to further detox your system while you increase fat burning.

Fats

Including another tablespoon of olive oil, in addition to what is in the cocktail, will keep you satisfied so you can better stave off hunger pains. The good fats are the most potent blood-sugar stabilizers.

Fruits

Berries, rich in fiber and flavonoids, combine with whey protein to provide a high-volume snack, on Days 4 and 5, so you won't be tempted to overeat at later meals.

YOU KNOW YOU ARE A FAT FLUSHER WHEN... you hug your partner and more than your belly touches.

Three Thermogenic Spices

Ginger, cinnamon, and dry mustard are spices that raise the body temperature, prompting your body to burn fat at an accelerated rate.

> *I tried the 5-Day Hot Metabolism Booster a week before an upcoming trip to New York City, knowing I would spend the weekend being tempted by the incredible foods the city has to offer. Not only did I drop four pounds and four inches, but I maintained these losses even after a weekend filled with sampling cuisines from all over the world!*
>
> —Linda, Fat Flush Fan

The Hot Metabolism Booster Cocktail

Makes 1 serving
1 large ripe tomato, or 8 ounces V8 or Knudsen's Very Veggie Juice

⅓ cup freshly squeezed lime or lemon juice	⅛ teaspoon cayenne (or as desired)
½ cup filtered water (unless using juice)	2 teaspoons olive oil
Handful of fresh parsley	½ teaspoon Seaweed Gomasio
Handful of fresh cilantro	½ teaspoon turmeric
1 green onion, chopped	1 teaspoon Flora-Key
1 clove garlic, crushed	1 tablespoon chia seeds
	6 ice cubes

Combine all the ingredients in a blender until the desired consistency is reached.

5-DAY HOT METABOLISM BOOSTER MEAL PLANNER

DAY 1

Breakfast
Hot Metabolism Booster Cocktail*

Snack
2 hard-boiled eggs with a pinch of dry
    mustard

Lunch
Turkey and Veggie Lettuce Wraps made
    with 4 ounces of sliced turkey, chopped
    cucumbers, tomatoes, and broccoli
    sprouts; 1 tablespoon each of olive oil
    and freshly squeezed lemon juice; and
    large lettuce leaves

Snack
Hot Metabolism Booster Cocktail*

Dinner
4 ounces grilled scallops with ginger and
    cayenne
1 cup each steamed yellow squash and
    zucchini with garlic

Before Bedtime
Hot Metabolism Booster Cocktail*

DAY 2

Breakfast
Hot Metabolism Booster Cocktail*

Snack
2 hard-boiled eggs with a pinch of garlic
    powder

Lunch
Chicken and Veggie Salad made with 4
    ounces of grilled chicken breast and
    cayenne, 1 tomato cut into wedges,
    broccoli and cauliflower florets, 1 table-
    spoon each of olive oil and freshly

squeezed lime juice, served over 2 cups
    of red leaf lettuce

Snack
Hot Metabolism Booster Cocktail*

Dinner
4 ounces grilled tilapia with freshly
    squeezed lemon juice and ginger
2 cups steamed spinach with garlic

Before Bedtime
Hot Metabolism Booster Cocktail*

DAY 3

Breakfast
Hot Metabolism Booster Cocktail*

Snack
2 hard-boiled eggs with a pinch of dry
    mustard

Lunch
Salmon Salad made with 4 ounces of
    canned salmon, chopped celery, 1
    tablespoon each of olive oil and freshly
    squeezed lemon juice, served over 2
    cups of mixed baby greens

Snack
Hot Metabolism Booster Cocktail*

Dinner
Grilled Shrimp and Veggie Kebob made
    with 4 ounces of shrimp, cherry
    tomatoes, and onion marinated in 2
    tablespoons of freshly squeezed lime
    juice plus ginger and cayenne
2 cups grilled eggplant with garlic

Before Bedtime
Hot Metabolism Booster Cocktail*

DAY 4

Breakfast
Hot Metabolism Booster Cocktail*
2 hard-boiled eggs with a pinch of
  cayenne

Snack
Strawberry Frappé made with 1 scoop of
  Fat Flush Vanilla Whey Protein or Fat
  Flush Body Protein, 6 large strawberries,
  1 cup of water, 1 teaspoon of Flora-Key,
  and 3 ice cubes

Lunch
Crab Salad Toss made with 4 ounces of
  crabmeat mixed with dry mustard, 1
  tomato, cut into wedges, 1 chopped
  green onion, 1 tablespoon each of

olive oil and freshly squeezed lemon
  juice, served over 2 cups of romaine
  lettuce

Snack
Hot Metabolism Booster Cocktail*

Dinner
Chicken and Veggie Stir-fry made with 4
  ounces of chicken and 1 cup each of
  snow peas and red bell peppers—stir-
  fry in ½ cup of chicken or veggie broth
  with ginger, ground cinnamon, and
  garlic

Before Bedtime
Hot Metabolism Booster Cocktail*

DAY 5

Breakfast
Hot Metabolism Booster Cocktail*
2 hard-boiled eggs with a pinch of garlic
  powder

Snack
Blueberry Frappé made with 1 scoop of Fat
  Flush Vanilla Whey Protein or Fat Flush
  Body Protein, 1 cup of blueberries, 1
  cup of water, 1 teaspoon of Flora-Key,
  and 3 ice cubes

Lunch
Tuna Stuffed Pepper made with 4 ounces
  of canned tuna, diced celery, and bell
  pepper with 1 tablespoon each of olive

oil and freshly squeezed lime juice,
  mounded into a large scooped-out bell
  pepper

Snack
Hot Metabolism Booster Cocktail*

Dinner
4 ounces grilled turkey burger made with
  dry mustard and cayenne, sliced red
  onion, and tomato slices
2 cups steamed kale with ginger and
  ground cinnamon

Before Bedtime
Hot Metabolism Booster Cocktail*

RESOURCES

Information is knowledge.

—Albert Einstein

Online Support

The Official Fat Flush for Life Web site
www.FatFlush.com

Fat Flush For Life Forum
www.annlouise.com/forum
Visit the Forum on my Web site,

created especially for my online community. Updates to the program as well as my blog are located here. This is also where you can also connect with other Fat Flushers and share success stories and tips to follow year round.

Fat Flush for Life General Resources

UNI KEY Health Systems
181 West Commerce Drive
Hayden Lake, ID 83835
1-800-888-4353
unikey@unkeyhealth.com
www.unikeyhealth.com
Here's my official distributor for many supplies and special test kits.

- Fat Flush Kit, which includes a thirty-day supply of Dieters' Multivitamin and Mineral, GLA-90, and the Weight Loss Formula
- CLA
- Flaxseed oil and softgels
- Fish oil and softgels
- Liver-Lovin' Formula
- Omega3 Chia Seeds
- Flora-Key
- Y-C Cleanse
- Fat Flush Body Protein
- Fat Flush Whey Protein
- Dr. Ohhira's Probiotic 12 Plus
- Dandelion Root Tea
- Stevia Plus
- BPA-free 1 Liter or 2.2 Liter Cran-water Bottle

To complement your detox journey, the following do-it-yourself tests are also available from UNI KEY. These include:
Tissue Mineral Analysis—This test

uses a small sample of hair cut from the back of your head. This analysis includes a full report, up to twenty pages, which graphically shows the levels of thirty-two major minerals and six toxic metals in the body. Each mineral is fully evaluated in terms of its relationship with other minerals, which is a key to glandular function and metabolism rate. This report provides information on the effect of vitamin deficits and excesses. There is also a complete discussion regarding environmental influences and disease tendencies based upon mineral levels and ratios. A list of recommended food choices and supplements, based upon the individual findings, is included at the end of the report. For further assistance, contacting Liz@annlouise.com can help you evaluate the findings for a modest fee.

Salivary Hormone Test—Unlike blood tests, which do not measure bio-available hormone activity, saliva testing is considered to be the most accurate measure of free, bio-available hormonal activity. This Personal Hormone Evaluation can be used to profile up to six hormones: estradiol, estriol, progesterone, testosterone, DHEA, and cortisol. Your personal results and a personal letter of recommendation from my office are mailed directly to your home.

Iodine Loading Test—The 24-hour iodine loading test is one of the best ways to gauge iodine levels. You will be provided with a kit and a letter of recommendation from my office.

Ranch Foods Direct

1-866-866-MEAT (6328)
www.ranchfoodsdirect.com
Ranch Foods Direct is a specialty meat company selling natural beef, raised without hormones or antibiotics, along with natural poultry, buffalo, eggs, cheese, pork, lamb, seafood, and many other high-quality food items. Rancher Mike Callicrate opened the Colorado Springs business in 2003 to combine the best of traditional animal husbandry practices with an innovative processing method that rinses the blood from the meat during processing, resulting in tender and more healthful meat. I have arranged a special offer for you to receive a discount on all of Mike's products. Please visit the Web site and then call 1-866-866-6328 to make your selection. The special discount code is "ALG."

Linda Mitchell

Personalized Fitness Programs
lmitchell@annlouise.com
Cincinnati, Ohio
www.LindaLuFitness.com
Linda Mitchell is an AFAA-certified personal trainer with twenty-five years' experience as a group exercise director in the fitness industry. Linda is a very qualified trainer with a long list of fitness titles to her credit. She currently teaches her own Bikini Boot Camp and specializes in designing fitness programs for people of all ages. She has been featured in several national magazines and also writes her own regular column called "Fit over Forty" for *Ms. Fitness* magazine. Linda will be glad to help you with all of your Fat Flush Fitness needs; you can catch her daily at www.annlouise.com.

Linda Shapiro

Personal Meal Planning Services
Naples, FL
LShapiro@annlouise.com
These days, maintaining a healthy eating lifestyle takes commitment as we struggle to balance our time between work, family, and personal obligations. Linda Shapiro, the recipe moderator on www.annlouise.com/forum, can help by providing personalized meal analysis and meal planning services for all of my programs, including Fat Flush for Life. Whether you need food shopping and meal preparation tips, your daily meal plans analyzed, or even customized menu planning, she is available for you.

Linda Hooper

Personalized Whole Health
Santa Fe, NM
1-480-688-3322
linda@lindahooper.com
For the past twenty years, Linda Hooper's international practice has embraced multidimensional approaches, including traditional Chinese medicine theory, to help uncover underlying causes of physical and/or emotional blocks. With a degree in Asian healing modalities, Linda is currently studying depth psychology at Pacifica Graduate School in Santa Barbara and is writing her first book. I have recommended her services to hundreds of clients when there is a need for "holistic" healing of the body, mind, and spirit.

Fitness Equipment

ReboundAIR

American Institute of Reboundology, Inc.
520 South Commerce Drive
Orem, UT 84058
1-888-464-5867
www.ReboundAir.com
Founded by Al Carter, the original pioneer of rebounding in this county, this company is one of the leaders in rebounder mini trampolines professionally designed and tested. With no assembly required, the ReboundAIR is portable and can be folded in half for easy transport. There is also a quarter-fold ReboundAIR available that is even more convenient for airline travelers, with a custom-fitted carry case and a free-pull dolly. This model has been tested on 300-pound individuals and is guaranteed for individuals up to 400 pounds. The lifetime warranty comes with a free wear-and-tear replacement. The stabilizing bar is sold separately and can be fitted with any model. Mention *Fat Flush for Life* when you call.

Needak Manufacturing

P.O. Box 776
O'Neill, NE 68763
1-800-232-5762
NeedakSales@NeedakRebounders.com
www.NeedakRebounders.com
Founded in 1990, this company is the only company that actually manufactures its own rebounders, right here in the United States. The Needak Soft-Bounce is the best-selling model for at home use. The company also offers folding travel rebounders for easy packing in a car trunk. The stabilizing bar is optional for those individuals who desire more balancing support. Mention *Fat Flush for Life* when you call.

Health Essentials

4607 Lakeview Canyon Road, Suite 101
Westlake Village, CA 91361
1-800-653-8881
DianeAddison@aol.com
www.HealthEssentials4you.com
The Lympholine has been scientifically designed to become the missing lymphatic pump that supports detoxification. Unlike a traditional trampoline, with a rigid frame and steel post legs, the Lympholine, has a full suspension system (similar to that of a car) with spring loaded legs, a flexing frame, and music wire springs that will absorb all of the harmful impact on your skeletal system. Bouncing on well-constructed, poorly designed rebounders may actually be harmful to one's muscles, joints, and nerves, but the Lympholine allows you to "float" and exercise at the same time. The Lympholine Rebounder includes a safety hand rail, spring cover, and an instructional DVD. Mention *Fat Flush for Life* when you call.

Fitness Wholesale

895 Hampshire Rd #A
Cuyahoga Falls, OH 44224
1-800-537-5512
www.fitnesswholesale.com
In addition to the full line of Thera-Band and Challenge PRO products, Fitness Wholesale supplies a full line of fitness equipment accessories: a variety of fitness balls, resistance bands and tubing, weights, mats, balance aids, and more.

Testing, Testing

ZRT Laboratory
  8605 SW Creekside Place
  Beaverton, OR 97008
  1-503-466-2445
  info@zrtlab.com
  www.zrtlab.com
  ZRT's new Vitamin D test uses state-of-the-art testing methodology to detect deficiencies in vitamin D as a potential cause of health problems. The vitamin D test spot-detects deficiencies in vitamin D (independently monitoring both vitamin D_2 and D_3 status) in your blood, as a potential cause of health problems ranging from osteoporosis to cardiovascular disease.

Educational Resources

American College of Nutrition
  300 S. Duncan Avenue, Suite 225
  Clearwater, FL 33755
  1-727-446-6086
  office@am-coll-nutr.org
  The American College of Nutrition was established in 1959 to promote scientific endeavor in the field of nutritional sciences.

Clayton College of Natural Health
  2140 11th Avenue South, Suite 305
  Birmingham, Alabama 35205
  1–800–659–2426
  communications@ccnh.edu
  www.ccnh.edu
  Clayton College offers college degree programs in natural health and holistic nutrition through distance education. These programs are designed to provide students with a wide variety of tools with which they can educate others in achieving and maintaining health through the use of natural elements such as proper diet, pure water, clean air, exercise, and rest. In addition, CCNH offers certificate programs in herbal studies, iridology, health care professional, and companion animal studies.

The National Institute of Whole Health
  Fraser Medical Complex
  326 Washington Street Annex
  Wellesley Hills, Massachusetts 02481
  1-888-354-4325
  info@wholehealtheducation.org
  The National Institute of Whole Health (NIWH) endeavors to provide curricula that approach health education training from a unique perspective. NIWH programs blend evidence-based medical science with a whole health perspective and holistic concepts of healing, unlike any traditional or alternative health school.

Must-Read Books

The Fat Flush Plan
  Ann Louise Gittleman, PhD, CNS
  McGraw-Hill (2002)
  The Fat Flush for Life provides the classic program that can be used in conjunction with *Fat Flush for Life*. A more stringent and regimented program, this book is ideal for individuals that need everything laid out on a daily basis in terms of food, exercise, sleep, and journaling.

The Fat Flush Cookbook
  Ann Louise Gittleman, PhD, CNS
  McGraw-Hill (2002)
  The Fat Flush Cookbook provides over two hundred recipes for breakfasts, snacks, lunches, dinners, desserts, and

beverages that are compatible with *Fat Flush for Life*.

Why Am I Always So Tired?
Ann Louise Gittleman, PhD, CNS
Harper San Francisco (1999)
This is the book that introduces the copper connection to a variety of health conditions, including weight loss, fatigue, anxiety, and hormonal imbalance.

Iodine: Why You Need It, Why You Can't Live Without It
Dr. David Brownstein
Medical Alternatives Press; 2nd edition (2006)
This book provides information on how iodine therapy is the missing link to today's health concerns.

The Power of 4: Your Ultimate Guide Guaranteed to Change Your Body and Transform Your Life
Paula Owens
Paula Owens; 2nd edition (2008)

This book is all-inclusive with the four pillars of health: holistic nutrition, lifestyle, exercise, and dietary supplements all in one.

Oil Pulling Therapy: Detoxifying and Healing the Body Through Oral Cleansing
Bruce Fife
Piccadilly Books, Ltd. (2008)
This book combines a revolutionary new treatment with the wisdom of Ayurvedic and modern science.

Diagnosis: Mercury: Money, Politics, and Poison
Jane M. Hightower, MD
Island Press; 1 edition (2008)
Throughout this book, Dr Hightower shows how important it is to understand mercury's wide-ranging health effects. She suggests there is an urgent need to set stricter limits on the amount of this neurotoxin emitted from coal-fired power plants, which contaminates the fish we eat.

Magazines

First for Women Magazine
270 Sylvan Avenue
Englewood Cliffs, NJ 07632
1-800-938-8312
www.firstforwomen.com
First For Women speaks directly to women about their real-life needs, concerns, and interests. You can also read my monthly advice column, "Nutrition Answers."

Totalhealth for Longevity Magazine
165 North 100 East, Suite 2
St. George, UT 84770-9963
1-888-316-6051
www.totalhealthmagazine.com
Totalhealth for Longevity is a comprehensive voice in antiaging, longevity, and self-managed natural health. Lyle Hurd, publisher extraordinaire, strives

to bring readers fresh new information and perspectives on all phases of longevity medicine so that you can make and educated decision on the quality of your life today…and tomorrow.

Taste for Life Magazine
86 Elm Street
Peterborough, NH 03458
1-603-924-7271
www.tasteforlife.com
Taste for Life is the fastest-growing, instore magazine for health food stores, natural product chains, food co-ops, and supermarkets nationwide. Its excellent articles on pertinent health issues offer readers an informative educational source on a variety of levels, including physical fitness. I sit on *Taste For Life's* editorial board.

Newsletters

Health Sciences Institute
Healthier News, LLC
702 Cathedral Street
Baltimore, MD 21201
1-888-213-0764
hsiresearch@healthiernews.com
www.hsibaltimore.com
As a member of this institute's professional advisory panel, I can verify that this cutting-edge newsletter is devoted to presenting extraordinary products to its members before those products hit the marketplace. They were the first to break the Ultra H3 story—the extraordinary product for arthritis, depression, and antiaging. The Health Sciences Institute provides private access to hidden cures, powerful discoveries, breakthrough treatments, and advances in modern, underground medicine.

The Sinatra Health Report
Published by Healthy Directions, LLC
7811 Montrose Road
Potomac, MD 20854
1-800-211-7643
www.drsinatra.com
Stephen Sinatra, MD, FACN, CNS, is a board-certified cardiologist and certified bioenergetic analyst with more than twenty years' experience in helping patients prevent and reverse heart disease. *The Sinatra Health Report* is published monthly by Phillips Health. Dr. Sinatra, to his credit, is a big proponent of detoxification and many of his newsletters discuss current research in the environmental medicine arena.

The Women's Health Letter
P.O. Box 467939

Atlanta, GA 31146-7939
1-800-728-2288
www.womenshealthletter.com
Nan Kathryn Fuchs, PhD, is the editor and my favorite nutritionist. Her comments regarding health, nutrition, and medicine as they relate to women are always on target.

Nutrition News
4108 Watkins Drive
Riverside, CA 92507
1-800-784-7550
www.nutritionnews.com
Siri Khalsa is a wonderful veteran journalist who has been in the business of providing health education for over twenty-five years. Her easy-to-read newsletter covers a wide variety of contemporary and current topics. It is distributed in health food stores through out the country, but you can subscribe directly.

Dr. Jonathan V. Wright's Nutrition & Healing
Healthier News, LLC
702 Cathedral Street
Baltimore, MD 21201
1-888-233-3402
www.wrightnewsletter.com
Nutrition and Healing is dedicated to helping you keep yourself and your family healthy by the safest and most effective means possible. Every month, you'll get information about diet, vitamins, minerals, herbs, natural hormones, natural energies, and other substances and techniques to prevent and heal illness, while prolonging your healthy life span.

Web Sites

Huggins Applied Healing
www.hugginsappliedhealing.com
Since 1973 Dr. Hal Huggins has been providing solutions for mercury toxicity. Many people have been told their health problems are all in their head

because their symptoms or diseases have no medically known cause or treatment. Dr. Huggins has discovered that dental toxicity due to mercury in amalgam fillings is the cause of many of these unexplained diseases and symptoms. Other standard dental practices such as root canals and implants have also been shown to contribute to many health issues that the medical community has no explanation for.

Gluten Free Travel, LLC

www.glutenfreetravelsite.com
GlutenFreeTravelSite.com was launched in April 2008 to help users quickly and easily access peer-written reviews of restaurants, hotels/resorts, cruise ships, and grocery stores around the world that cater to the gluten-free community. The site is organized by geographic region to make submitting and searching reviews very user-friendly. The site has recently added a major new section called "Gluten Free Restaurant Menus" to its Web site, at www.glutenfreetravelsite.com/restaurants. Designed to help people on a gluten-free diet find national and regional restaurants that offer gluten-free items on their menu, this new part of the Web site also lists restaurants that have taken the time to accommodate the fast-growing celiac community.

Environmental Working Group

www.ewg.org
The mission of the Environmental Working Group (EWG) is to use the power of public information to protect public health and the environment.

AromaCafé

www.myaromacafe.net
AromaCafé provides unsurpassed quality and purity in essential oils. Every batch is fully GC/MS tested and they offer single oils as well as blends.

Home Saunas

EZe Saunas

www.ezesauna.com
In 1983, EZe Saunas introduced the Far-Infrared Sauna Systems in the United States to promote comfort and healing. Recently the company introduced their internationally patented Micro-Carbon Fiber Flat Heaters.

Sunlight Saunas

www.sunlightsaunas.com
Founded in 1999, Sunlight Saunas produces and sells far infrared saunas for therapeutic benefit for both residential and commercial use.

MPS Global

www.mpsglobal.us
Although it looks like an ordinary infrared sauna, the Management of Personal Health System (MPS) sauna uses active carbon fibers that cover most of the interior within the sauna and boasts the largest radiation surface area in the industry.

NOTES

CHAPTER 1

1   A. Ellin, "Flush Those Toxins! Eh, Not So Fast," *New York Times* (January 22, 2009).
2   "Oxygen Radical Absorbance Capacity of Selected Foods," USDA (November 2007).
3   J. F. Colombel, A. J. M. Watson, and M. F. Neurath, "The 10 Remaining Mysteries of Inflammatory Bowel Disease," *Gut* 57 (2008): 429–33.
4   H. J. Van Kruiningen and J. F. Colombel, "The Forgotten Role of Lymphangitis in Crohn's Disease," *Gut* 57 (2008): 1–4.
5   W. D. van Marken Lichtenbelt, J. W. Vanhommerig, N. M. Smulders, J. M. Drossaerts, G. J. Kemerink, N. D. Bouvy, P. Schrauwen, and G. J. Teule, "Cold-Activated Brown Adipose Tissue in Healthy Men," *New England Journal of Medicine* 360, no. 15 (April 9, 2009): 1500–1508.
6   A. M. Cypess, S. Lehman, G. Williams, I. Tal, D. Rodman, A. B. Goldfine, F. C. Kuo, E. L. Palmer, Y. H. Tseng, A. Doria, G. M. Kolodny, and C. R. Kahn, "Identification and Importance of Brown Adipose Tissue in Adult Humans," *New England Journal of Medicine* 360, no. 15 (April 9, 2009): 1509–17.
7   David F. Horrobin, MD, PhD, *Clinical Uses of Essential Fatty Acids* (Montreal-London: Eden Press, 1982); Horrobin, "The Regulation of Prostaglandins Biosynthesis by the Manipulation of Essential Fatty Acids Metabolism." *Review of Drug Metabolism and Drug Interaction* 4 (1983): 339.
8   Ide Takashi, Masayo Kushiro, and Yoko Takahashi, "Dietary Mold Oil Rich in Gamma Linolenic Acid Increases Insulin-Dependent Glucose Utilization in Isolated Rat Adipocytes," Laboratory of Nutrition Biochemistry, National Food Research Institute, 2-1-12 Kannondai, Tsukuba Science City, Ibaraki 305–8642, Japan.
9   A. D'Almeida, J. P. Carter, A. Anatol, and C. Prost, "Effects of a Combination of Evening Primrose Oil (Gamma Linolenic Acid) and Fish Oil (Eicosapentaenoic + Docahexaenoic Acid) versus Magnesium, and versus Placebo in Preventing Preeclampsia," *Women's Health* 19, nos. 2–3 (1992): 117–131.
10 U. Risérus, L. Berglund, and B. Vessby, "Conjugated Linoleic Acid (CLA) Reduced Abdominal Adipose Tissue in Obese Middle-Aged Men with Signs of the Metabolic Syndrome: A Randomized Controlled Trial," *International Journal of Obesity* 25 (2001): 1129–35.
11 J. A. Paniagua, A. Gallego de la Sacristana, I. Romero, A. Vidal-Puig, J. M. Latre, E. Sanchez, P. Perez-Martinez, J. Lopez-Miranda, and F. Perez-Jimenez, "Monounsaturated Fat–Rich Diet Prevents Central Body Fat Distribution and Decreases Postprandial Adiponectin Expression Induced by a Carbohydrate-Rich Diet in Insulin-Resistant Subjects," *Diabetes Care* 30: 1717–23; published online before print as 10.2337/dc06–2220.
12 ATS 2006 International Conference: Abstract C88. Presented May 23, 2006.
13 Eve Van Cauter, PhD, Rachel Leproult, MS, and Laurence Plat, MD, "Age-Related Changes in Slow Wave Sleep and REM Sleep and Relationship with Growth Hormone and Cortisol Levels in Healthy Men," *Journal of the American Medical Association*, no. 284 (2000): 861–68.
14 National Sleep Foundation, "Sleep in America Poll, 2001–2002," Washington, DC: National Sleep Foundation.
15 H. Kather and B. Simon, "Opioid Peptides and Obesity," *Lancet* 2 (1979): 905.
16 M. Rosenbaum, R. L. Leibel, and J. Hirsh, "Medical Progress: Obesity," *New England Journal of Medicine* 337 (1997): 396–407.

CHAPTER 2

1   R. E. Ley, P. J. Turnbaugh, S. Klein, and J. I. Gordon, "Microbial Ecology: Human Gut Microbes Associated with Obesity," *Nature* 444, no. 7122 (2006): 1022–23.
2   Ibid.
3   P. J. Turnbaugh, R. E. Ley, M. A. Mahowald, V. Magrini, E. R. Mardis, and J. I. Gordon, "An Obesity-Associated Gut Microbiome with Increased Capacity for Energy Harvest," *Nature* 444, no. 7122 (2006): 1027–31.
4   Alison M. Hill, Jonathan D. Buckley, Karen J. Murphy, and Peter R. C. Howe, "Combining Fish-Oil Supplements with Regular Aerobic Exercise Improves Body Composition and Cardiovascular Disease Risk Factors," *American Journal of Clinical Nutrition* 85 (May 2007): 1267–74.
5   Dr. Stephen Sinatra, *Heart, Health & Nutrition* newsletter (March 2006): 2, published by Healthy Directions, Potomac, MD.
6   Guy E. Abraham, MD, "Facts about Iodine and Autoimmune Thyroiditis," *Original Internist* 15, no. 2 (June 2008): 75–76; Abraham and David Brownstein, MD, "A Simple Procedure Combining the Evaluation of Whole Body Sufficiency for Iodine with the Efficiency of the Body to Utilize Peripheral Iodide: The Triple Test," *Original Internist* 14, no. 1 (March 2007): 17–23; Abraham, Brownstein, and J. D. Flechas, "The Saliva/

Serum Iodide Ratio as an Index of Sodium/Iodide Symporter Efficiency," *Original Internist* 12, no. 4 (2005): 152–56.

7   Nan Kathryn Fuchs, PhD, ed., *Women's Health Letter,* 1-800-728-2288, Women's Health, P.O. Box 467939, Atlanta, GA 31146–7939.

CHAPTER 4

1   M. Voevodin, A. Sinclair, R. Gibson, et al., "The Effect of CLA on Body Composition in Humans: Systematic Review and Meta-Analysis," *Asia Pacific Journal of Clinical Nutrition* 14 (2005): S55.
2   S. Baxter, E. Shaw, and A. M. Minihane, *Health Benefits of Organic Food: Effects of the Environment,* ed. D. I. Givens (Reading, UK: University of Reading, 2008).

CHAPTER 6

1   S. E. Taylor, L. C. Klein, B. P. Lewis, T. L. Gruenewald, R. A. R. Gurung, and J. A. Upsedegraff, "Female Responses to Stress: Tend and Befriend, Not Fight or Flight," *Psychological Review* 107, no. 3 (2000): 41–429.

CHAPTER 7

1   S. B. Sisson, P. T. Katzmarzyk, C. P. Earnest, C. Bouchard, S. N. Blair, and T. S. Church, "Volume of Exercise and Fitness Nonresponse in Sedentary, Postmenopausal Women," *Medicine and Science in Sports and Exercise* 41, no. 3 (2009): 539–45.
2   A. Bhattacharya, E. P. McCutcheon, E. Shvartz, and J. E. Greenleaf, "Body Acceleration Distribution and O_2 Uptake in Humans during Running and Jumping," *Journal of Applied Physiology* 49 (1980): 881–87.

CHAPTER 8

1   H. W. Cohen, MD, and H. D. Sesso, ScD, MPH, "Low-Salt Diet May Not Be Best for Heart," *Journal of General Internal Medicine* [cited 2008 May 15]. Available from http://healthlibrary. brighamandwomens.org/RelatedItems/6,615802.

CHAPTER 9

1   H. V. Amith, Anil V. Ankola, L. Nagesh, "Effect of Oil Pulling on Plaque and Gingivitis," *Journal of Oral Health and Community Dentistry* 1, no. 1 (January 2007): 12–18.
2   Ibid.
3   B. Fife, *Oil Pulling Therapy: Detoxifying and Healing the Body Through Oral Cleansing* (Colorado Springs, CO: Piccadilly Books, 2008).

CHAPTER 13

1   *British Medical Journal,* "Maintaining Aerobic Fitness Could Delay Biological Aging by up to 12 Years, Study Shows," *ScienceDaily* (April 10, 2008), accessed July 27 2009, http://www.sciencedaily.com/releases/2008/04/080409205827.htm.

CHAPTER 17

1   F. M. Sacks, G. A. Bray, V. J. Carey, S. R. Smith, D. H. Ryan, S. D. Anton, K. McManus, C. M. Champagne, L. M. Bishop, N. Laranjo, M. S. Leboff, J. C. Rood, L. de Jonge, C. M. Loria, E. Obarzanek, and D. A. Williamson, "Randomized Trial Comparing Fat, Protein, and Carbohydrate Composition of Diets for Weight Loss for Two Years," *New England Journal of Medicine* 360, no. 9 (February 26, 2009).
2   A. K. Kant, M. B. Andon, T. J. Angelopoulos, and J. M. Rippe, "Association of Breakfast Energy Density with Diet Quality and Body Mass in American Adults: National Health and Nutrition Examination Surveys, 1999–2004," *American Journal of Clinical Nutrition* 88 (2008): 1396–1404.

APPENDIX

1   J. E. Flood and B. J. Rolls, "Soup Preloads in a Variety of Forms Reduce Meal Energy Intake," *Appetite* 49 no. 3 (2007): 626–34.

2   M. S. Chi, E. T. Koh, and T. J. Stewart, "Effects of Garlic on Lipid Metabolism in Rats Fed Cholesterol or Lard," Departments of Home Economics and Chemistry, Alcorn State University, Lorman, MS 39096.

3   T. A. Mori, et al., "Dietary Fish as a Major Component of a Weight-loss Diet: Effect on Serum Lipids, Glucose, and Insulin Metabolism in Overweight Hypertensive Subjects," *American Journal of Clinical Nutrition* 70 (November 1999): 817–25.

4   G. Jiang and B. B. Zhang, *American Journal of Physiology-Endocrinology and Metabolism* 284, no. 4: E671.

INDEX